Consulting in a Nutshell

Praise for the first edition:

'…a unique book, written by a unique GP. There is no one better placed to pull together decades of learning and experience on how to achieve the greatest success in the general practice consultation. The relaxed pace of writing, the accessible examples, the clear narrative and the engaging anecdotes make this a resource that is accessible and useful to all who seek to improve their clinical consulting skills.'

Helen Stokes-Lampard, former Chair of the Royal College of General Practitioners

'Excellent and easy to remember structure; this is the approach I'll use daily.'

GP ST3

The second edition of this well-received book, fully revised to reflect changes to the RCGP Membership examination, helps GPs establish ways of thinking, talking and behaving in the consultation that are most likely to lead to good outcomes. It describes a simple three-part approach to the consultation's essential task, which is to convert a patient's problem into a plan acceptable to both patient and doctor. It combines reader-friendly explanations, helpful illustrations and examples from everyday practice.

Consulting in a Nutshell will help GPs at every career stage – from medical student to SCA candidate to experienced practitioner – to analyse, develop and grow their personal consulting style. At a time of ongoing and profound change in primary care, it aims to ensure that seeing patients and having good consultations becomes and remains a source of satisfaction and fulfilment.

T0260283

Consulting in a Nutshell

A practical guide to successful general practice consultations before, during and beyond the MRCGP

Second Edition

Roger Neighbour
OBE MA MB BChir DSc FRCP FRCGP FRACGP

Illustrations by Jamie Hynes
MB ChB FRCGP DRCOG PGCertMedEd

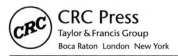

CRC Press
Taylor & Francis Group
Boca Raton London New York

CRC Press is an imprint of the
Taylor & Francis Group, an **informa** business

Second edition published 2024
by CRC Press
2385 NW Executive Center Drive, Suite 320, Boca Raton, FL 33431

and by CRC Press
4 Park Square, Milton Park, Abingdon, Oxon, OX14 4RN

CRC Press is an imprint of Taylor & Francis Group, LLC

© 2024 Roger Neighbour

First Edition published in 2021

ISBN: 978-1-032-61917-0 (hbk)
ISBN: 978-1-032-61089-4 (pbk)
ISBN: 978-1-032-61920-0 (ebk)

DOI: 10.1201/9781032619200

Typeset in Bembo
by KnowledgeWorks Global Ltd.

The most important thing is to find out what is the most important thing.

Zen Master Shunryu Suzuki (1904–1971)

It is more important to know what patient has the disease than what disease the patient has.

Variously attributed to Hippocrates (c. 460–370 BCE) or Sir Wiliam Osler (1849–1919)

Examinations are formidable even to the best prepared, for the greatest fool may ask more than the wisest man can answer.

Charles Caleb Colton (1780–1832)

I offer this book with affection, admiration and gratitude to

Jan-Helge Larsen FRCGP of Copenhagen,

a fine doctor, a great opener of doors and windows, and a good friend.

Contents

Foreword to the First Edition

Early during my professional general practitioner training, I bumped into a warm, friendly, unassuming GP at the RCGP Headquarters in Princes Gate, London. In our informal interaction, he swiftly put me at my ease, got to the heart of my concerns and made me feel valued. As he walked away, my companion (also a GP in training) said in an awed voice, 'You do realise that was the legendary Roger Neighbour?' ... Two decades later, I am honoured to be asked to write this Foreword to a new book that brings together the collected wisdom of a man whose work and example have guided my thinking, shaped my practice and reinforced my professionalism.

The clinical consultation is undoubtedly an art form like playing the piano, and any skill requires many, many hours of practice. Whilst few ever truly master a musical instrument, most doctors who are selected to train in general practice can become experts – but we continue to learn through our entire careers, and we each develop our own style.

Consulting in a Nutshell is a unique book, written by a unique GP. There is no one better placed to pull together decades of learning and experience on how to achieve the greatest success in the general practice consultation. The relaxed pace of writing, the accessible examples, the clear narrative and the engaging anecdotes make this a resource that is accessible and useful to all who seek to improve their clinical consulting skills.

Having seen so many trainees get stuck in a rut when they prepare for examinations, I was pleased to see the section tackling head on the formulaic approach to consulting that some unfortunately develop. As one lovely example in the book illustrates, our patients are frequently very astute, and as such, any hint of being treated in a standardised way really irritates; the artificial application of the 'ideas, concerns and expectations' cliché tacked onto the end of a mediocre consultation being cited as how NOT to do it ('Don't ICE me!'). Other concepts covered include reiterating content through the use of receipts and the idea that a consultation is a conversation with a point.

Modern UK general practice is the cornerstone of an effective National Health Service and is respected worldwide. As reflective holistic practitioners, we are ever learning, ever seeking to improve; even the most experienced of us benefit from taking a step back, thinking about our style, our motivations and our impact. *Consulting in a Nutshell* is a superb companion for any clinician aspiring to be the best they can be – thank you, Roger Neighbour, our profession owes you so much.

Professor Helen Stokes-Lampard
PhD FRCGP DSc

Foreword to the Second Edition

General practice is the cornerstone of the NHS, helping over 50 million people and carrying out over 370 million consultations every year. The Royal College of General Practitioners (RCGP) is the professional membership body for GPs in the UK. Its purpose is to encourage, foster and maintain the highest possible standards in general medical practice. The College supports GPs through all stages of their career, from medical students considering general practice to training, qualified years and retirement. This new edition of *Consulting in a Nutshell* will support all aspiring and qualified GPs, whatever the stage of their professional journey.

In 1969, Dr Kenneth Lane famously described general practice as 'the longest art.' Just as art is a continuous process of exploration where more recent periods such as minimalism, photorealism and contemporary art grew out of surrealism, expressionism, Pop-Art and Arte Povera, so general practice evolves. The COVID-19 pandemic accelerated this evolution. It impacted both the demand for and provision of healthcare. As the first point of patient contact and the gateway to secondary care, general practice rapidly transformed and adapted. Remote consultations in primary care increased to provide care for COVID-19 and non–COVID-19 patients whilst protecting patients and healthcare professionals. In-person consultations also continued where necessary. General practice continued to provide care for patients when many other NHS services had to close down.

Inevitably, the pandemic also impacted the examination for Membership of the Royal College of General Practitioners (MRCGP), the UK's GP licensing assessment. The exam's tripos of Applied Knowledge Test (AKT), Workplace-Based Assessment (WPBA) and a Clinical Skills Assessment (CSA) was disrupted when, in March 2020, it became unsafe to continue delivering the CSA. The Recorded Consultation Assessment (RCA), developed in record time by a small, exceptionally dedicated team of examiners, proved to be a very reliable emergency replacement that has enabled many thousands of colleagues to complete their training and safely enter the GP workforce. The RCGP is now returning to a standardised Simulated Consultation Assessment (SCA) portraying the sorts of cases seen by GPs every day across the UK.

Roger Neighbour is to general practice what Dame Mary Berry is to baking, a national treasure! Few could construct a recipe that so perfectly balances two different but complementary flavours: SCA exam preparation and the skills required for a life-long career of successful general practice consulting thereafter. General practice is an art, but it is underpinned by science. *Consulting in a Nutshell* (Second Edition) provides all the necessary ingredients to support GP trainees preparing for the SCA, their trainers and all other GPs aspiring to further develop their patient-centredness. As a former President of the RCGP and an international expert on communication skills, no one is better placed to share with the reader the College's philosophy of *Cum scientia caritas*, science with compassion. Thank you, Roger, on behalf of general practice and the patients we serve.

Professor Rich Withnall
MD FRCP FRCP FAcadMEd SFFMLM

Preface to the First Edition

Thank you for reading this book. I wrote it out of a belief that a well-conducted consultation, combining kindness and competence, is one of the many small miracles that take place every day in Britain's GP surgeries. And I hope you'll agree that the world needs all the miracles it can get.

When the book was still at the 'idea' stage, the publishers, as is their normal practice, sent an outline and some sample chapters to various referees for their evaluation. Luckily, they all recommended publication; but some, having seen the subtitle, offered me a piece of advice. 'Make your mind up,' they said. 'Is it meant to be a practical manual for working GPs, or is it a *get-you-through-the-exam* crammer for trainees sitting the MRCGP?'

Either or: two of the most dispiriting words in the language; but also, if they become a challenge, two of the most energising. Why, I thought, should the way you consult under exam conditions, when you're on your best behaviour and trying to showcase your skills, need to be any different from what you would aspire to do on good days and bad days alike in the hurly-burly of everyday practice? So I've stuck to my guns and tried to make what follows equally relevant to medical students and junior doctors wanting to get into good habits; to MRCGP candidates motivated partly by the fear of failure; and to established GPs hoping to keep their consulting skills resilient under real-world pressure. If you're in this last category, please be patient when my text at times is aimed specifically at the younger groups. Show them the same courtesy and consideration you would when you find yourself behind a learner driver on the road. And, to continue the analogy, isn't it sometimes the case that seeing a driver under instruction signalling *left* in textbook fashion when exiting a roundabout serves as a timely reminder of how easy it is to let one's own high standards slip?

As I write, British general practice is in danger of being brought to its knees for lack of manpower and resources, and is likely to remain so for a considerable time[1]. Some commentators assert that, under siege conditions, we should enter survival mode and dispense with patient-centred consulting as an outdated luxury. I profoundly disagree. The best way to keep alive in an ice age is to not let the fire that warms you go out. Numerous colleagues tell me that consulting in a way they can be proud of is their best immunisation against the disillusionment and burnout of which our profession is currently at risk. The impact of bureaucracy, shortages and overwhelming demand is undeniable; but when the door closes and it's just you and the patient in the consulting room, getting the one-to-one part of the job right is never more important.

Roger Neighbour
Bedmond, Hertfordshire
April 2020

---

[1] Since I drafted this passage, the global COVID-19 pandemic has – temporarily, I hope – transformed general practice into a largely arm's length affair, with most consultations taking place by telephone or video.

Preface to the Second Edition

I have been very gratified by the feedback I've received on this book's first edition, particularly the response of its primary readership, young GPs preparing for the MRCGP exam, the turnstile that admits them to their future careers. They have confirmed my belief that what they (and lots of other GPs) needed, at a time of unprecedented pressure and turbulence in general practice, was a simple approach that would help them to consult competently, compassionately and time-efficiently, in a way that satisfied their patients, the examiners and them themselves. I particularly appreciated the message I had from one successful candidate who chortled a triumphant 'Wooohooo!'

Just before the first edition went to press, COVID-19 struck. The world changed forever, and general practice along with it. Traditional ways of working that had long been taken for granted had to be unceremoniously abandoned and replaced by ones where face-to-face human contact was a danger, not a comfort. Almost overnight, the proportion of GP consultations conducted over the phone rocketed from less than 10% to over 80%. In July 2020, Matt Hancock, then the Secretary of State for Health and Social Care, said in a speech to the Royal College of Physicians, 'From now on, all consultations should be teleconsultations unless there's a compelling clinical reason not to.' And he didn't mean just so long as the pandemic lasted.

Pre-pandemic, one component of the MRCGP exam was the Clinical Skills Assessment (CSA). Candidates would come to the RCGP headquarters in London and conduct a simulated surgery of 13 role-played patients, each accompanied by an examiner who would assess the doctor's decision-making and interpersonal skills. The social distancing rules imposed during lockdown, however, put an abrupt stop to the CSA, threatening to render an entire year's cohort of GP trainees unable to complete their training.

The response of the MRCGP examiners – and I take my hat off to them – was rapidly to develop an alternative 'contactless' exam, the Recorded Consultation Assessment (RCA). This required candidates to submit a portfolio of audio or video recordings of their own real-life consultations with actual patients, the majority of which took place over the telephone. These were subsequently reviewed and marked by examiners in much the same way as the CSA had been. It is a minor miracle of medical assessment that an entirely new module could be conceived, developed, validated, calibrated, approved by the General Medical Council (GMC) as an emergency licensing exam, and implemented on a national scale, all within a few weeks. For all its shortcomings, the RCA rescued the careers of literally thousands of young GPs.

As we now know, the restrictions on face-to-face consulting lasted much longer than had been anticipated at the start of the pandemic. General practice, for so long the natural home of doctors who enjoyed dealing with people, became a largely faceless exercise, the daily experience of GPs not much different from working in a telephone call centre. Their ability to interact with patients, to read their body language and examine them if necessary was severely compromised. GPs found themselves missing out on much of the subtlety, intimacy and personal connection they had hitherto enjoyed. And a much-vaunted advantage of remote consulting – that it made more efficient use of a doctor's time – proved to be an illusion. Many telephone consultations ended with the patient still having to attend the surgery to be examined, thus engendering two consultations where one would have done.

Patients weren't happy either. Although telephone consultations could be convenient for patients with minor problems and busy lives, many others, especially the elderly and the socially disadvantaged, keenly missed being able to 'see the doctor'. Relatively deserted surgery premises gave the false impression that GPs were idle, a calumny widely propagated in some quarters of the national press. GPs' esteem in the eyes of the public nosedived, to such an extent that Sajid Javid, Hancock's successor as Secretary of State, stood at the Despatch Box in the House of Commons on 14 September 2021 and declared, apparently unembarrassed by the U-turn, 'It is high time GPs offer face-to-face appointments to anyone who wants one.' As I write, in mid-2023, the pendulum that swings between 'remote is good' and 'face-to-face is best' is still in motion. It will probably settle somewhere in between, with general practice becoming a hybrid of about 60% in-person consultations, 30% remote (telephone or video) and 10% online e-consultations.

The RCA, too, outlived its usefulness. Essential under lockdown conditions though it was, as post-COVID general practice consulting gradually reverted to something like the *status quo ante*, its deficiencies as a method of assessment could no longer be overlooked. There were practical difficulties in obtaining the necessary consent from patients and in uploading recordings. In addition, candidates were often bewildered by having to choose suitable consultations to submit – ones that were neither too simple to showcase the necessary degree of clinical skill and judgement nor so challenging as to be impossible to complete in the 12 minutes allowed.

As the pandemic subsided, reinstating its predecessor, the CSA, would have made the MRCGP again vulnerable to disruption by the possible return of the virus or any future contingency with similar consequences for face-to-face consulting. So a new module, future-proofed against these threats, was developed – the Simulated Consultation Assessment (SCA). In devising the SCA, the College examiners consulted widely with stakeholders, including trainees, trainers, Deaneries, the Statutory Educational Bodies in England, Wales, Scotland and Northern Ireland, the Academy of Medical Royal Colleges, medical educationists, psychometricians and the GMC. The result is as accurate and dependable an assessment of general practice's soft skills as human endeavour can create.

After thorough piloting, the SCA came on stream in November 2023 and now sits alongside the other two components of the MRCGP exam, the Applied Knowledge Test (AKT) and the Workplace-Based Assessment (WPBA). It has been approved by the GMC as having the validity and reliability essential in a high-stakes licensing examination. In other words, it tests what it *needs* to test, and does so fairly, consistently and without bias.

The SCA consists of 12 simulated consultations, each lasting 12 minutes with a 3-minute break between them, conducted remotely via an online platform. It can only be taken during or after the third year (ST3) of GP vocational training. It is designed to assess a candidate's ability to integrate and apply clinical, professional and communication skills appropriate for safe, independent general practice in the UK. Since the selection of cases is determined by the examiners, not the candidate, the SCA is much easier to standardise and calibrate than the RCA and is thus inherently a fairer and more reliable assessment.

The 'patients' are professional role-players who are trained, calibrated and standardised so that, although the case presents in the same way to every candidate, it unfolds according to the approach of the individual doctor, as in real life. The cases are usually consultations with patients, or in some instances, their carer, partner, parent or another healthcare professional, reflecting the various situations a GP may be presented with in everyday practice, irrespective of the setting in which they work. The

SCA is delivered online, with candidates sitting the exam in their own or a local practice, so that they no longer suffer the inconvenience and expense of the trip to London that the CSA had entailed. In some SCA cases, doctor and patient will be visible to each other on video; in others, simulating a telephone consultation, only voices will be heard. The entire 'surgery' is recorded and uploaded onto a dedicated IT platform, to be marked later, each case by different examiners. Candidates are thus not distracted during their consultations by the presence, seen or unseen, of a third-party assessor.

Does the new format call for any change in how candidates should go about acquiring and consolidating their consulting skills? Absolutely *not*. In the SCA, as in its predecessors, success depends only on managing patients safely and reasonably, nothing more. It is not achieved by trying to game the system or by play-acting the role of 'good doctor' with formulaic phrases and stereotyped behavioural sub-routines. Neither does it require sticking slavishly to any particular consultation model, nor trying to do a hospital-style history and examination at breakneck speed. Candidates whose consultations have a securely embedded core structure, and who can adapt it appropriately to the singularities of each patient's situation, will pass. The best way to prepare for the SCA is to learn good consulting habits early in your training, practise them in your surgeries over the weeks and months until they become second nature – and then, on the day of the exam, just do what you *always* do.

In this new edition of *Consulting in a Nutshell*, I have updated the text to take account of the new SCA module. An Addendum (*Reassurance to SCA candidates*) makes explicit how the approach described in this book maps onto what the SCA examiners are looking for and how it is marked. A series of 'EXAM POINT' boxes in the text expand on issues of particular relevance to SCA candidates. I have also incorporated some of the lessons learned during the pandemic into the sections on remote consulting, which is destined to remain a more prominent feature of general practice than it was before.

Roger Neighbour
Bedmond, Hertfordshire

Addendum – Reassurance to SCA candidates (and their teachers)

Ideally, if you're preparing to sit the Simulated Consultation Assessment (SCA) of the MRCGP exam, I'd like you to read or re-read this Addendum after you've finished Chapter 3 of this book. Why? By then, you'll have a good overview of the consultation structure I'm advocating. But you'll probably be wondering whether reading this or any other book can really help you to pass an exam where it's your behaviour and your thought processes, not just your knowledge, that are being assessed. And I want to reassure you; most of what medical educators commonly refer to as 'consulting skills' are *already* in your repertoire. You've already acquired them in the course of your family and social life, talking and interacting with people whom you care about.

Essentially, the general practice consultation is just having a conversation with another person, and you already know how to do that. The only difference is that the consultation is a conversation *with a point* – the point being to help your patient to solve a problem. What this book will do is give you a basic problem-solving structure for your consultations, plus a few simple strategies, onto which you can peg your existing communication skills in order for you to be as helpful as possible to your patient.

The consultation, whether in real life or in the SCA, is not a circus act where you are expected to show off your repertoire of consulting 'tricks' in order to win the applause of the audience. The examiner is not marking your consultation according to a checklist, ticking off *ICE? Summarise? Open questions? Smoking history? Options offered?* And you won't gain marks just for coming out with a few jargon phrases or formulaic questions. Your patients and your examiners are not overly bothered about *how* you deliver good, safe care – the only thing that matters is that, one way or another, you *do*.

We can learn a lot about what the SCA examiners *are* looking for, and what sorts of things they mark down, from the information the College publishes about how cases are marked and from the feedback comments provided to candidates.

The purpose of the SCA[2] is to assess your ability to integrate and apply your clinical, professional and communication skills, demonstrating that you can achieve the principles underlying GMC's *Good Medical Practice*, i.e. that:

- your patients are kept safe;
- you can be adaptable in treating different types of patients and illnesses;
- you can manage risk, medical complexity and uncertainty; and
- you show appropriate behaviours, attitudes and concerns for your patients.

Each SCA case is marked in three separate domains:

- *Data gathering and diagnosis* (DG&D), i.e. finding out what the patient's problem is
- *Clinical management and medical complexity* (CM&C), i.e. working out what to do about the problem
- *Relating to others* (RTO) i.e. conducting the consultation in an effective, considerate, respectful and professional manner

For each domain, the examiner will award you one of four possible grades:

- *Clear pass* (earning 3 marks), indicating that you clearly meet the standard expected of a safe and independent newly-qualified GP
- *Pass* (2 marks), indicating that, despite some minor errors or omissions, your performance was generally good and you are fit to practise unsupervised
- *Fail* (1 mark), indicating that, although you presented some evidence of competence, it was too insubstantial or incomplete for you to be allowed to practise unsupervised

---

[2] These and other factual details of the SCA in this book are accurate at the time of writing. However, the RCGP website should be regarded as the only 'single point of truth' for reliable and up-to-date information. MRCGP candidates and their teachers should always refer to the relevant sections of the website.

- *Clear fail* (0 marks), indicating that only minimal evidence of competence was presented, or that you put the patient in danger

In deciding their grades, examiners are guided by the following general descriptors of the standard required to pass in each domain:

Data gathering and diagnosis:

- The candidate systematically gathers and organises relevant and targeted information to address the needs of the patient and their problem(s).
- The candidate adopts a structured and informed approach to problem-solving, generating an appropriate differential diagnosis or relying on first principles where the presentation is undifferentiated, uncertain, or complex.

Note some of the key words in this description – *systematically* gathers ... *relevant* and *targeted* information. They want to see that you have a degree of organisation in how you set about discovering the problem, and that you can tell the difference between information that matters and information that does not. If the nature of the problem isn't immediately clear, they want to know that you have some strategies for coping with the uncertainty.

Clinical management and medical complexity:

- The candidate demonstrates the ability to formulate safe and appropriate management options, which include effective prioritisation, continuity and time and self-management.
- The candidate demonstrates commitment to providing optimum care in the short and long term, whilst acknowledging the challenges.

The examiners are all GPs who live and work in the same real world as you. They know that time is short, resources are limited, and that you may have to prioritise some aspects of management over others. But they expect you, nevertheless, to do your best to ensure your patients get the best possible care.

Relating to others:

- The candidate demonstrates ethical awareness.
- The candidate shows the ability to communicate in a person–centred way.
- The candidate demonstrates initiative and flexibility in using various consultation approaches in order to overcome any communication barriers and reach a shared understanding with the patient.

Behind the formal wording of this description lie some basic principles of human interaction – try to understand the other person's situation, respect their point of view, and treat them as you yourself would wish to be treated. It is also clear that the examiners are not expecting you to stick rigidly to any particular consultation model, but rather to be able to adapt your approach to whatever works best for the individual patient.

All SCA candidates, whether or not they are successful overall, receive feedback about every domain in every case for which they are graded *Fail* or *Clear Fail*. The examiners have a fixed range of feedback statements available to them in all three marking domains and for their overarching reflections, and they select which, if any, apply in the case they have been marking. The feedback statements are necessarily couched in critical language describing poor performance, but we can easily infer from them the types of behaviour that examiners regard as desirable. The feedback statements (taken *verbatim* from the RCGP's SCA webpages) are as follows:

Data gathering and diagnosis:

- Data was insufficient to enable a safe assessment of the condition/ situation.
- Existing information about the case was insufficiently utilised.
- Relevant psychological or social information was inadequately or inappropriately recognised or responded to.
- Data gathering was unsystematic and/or disorganised.
- Ineffective approach or prioritisation in data gathering when presented with multiple or complex problems.
- The implications of relevant findings identified during the data gathering were insufficiently recognised or understood.
- Differential diagnoses or hypotheses were inadequately generated or tested.
- Decision-making or the diagnosis was illogical, incorrect or incomplete.

Clinical management and medical complexity:

- The management plan relating to referrals was inappropriate or not reflective of current practice.
- The management plan relating to the prescribing of medication was inappropriate or not reflective of current practice.
- The management plan relating to investigations was inappropriate or not reflective of current practice.

- The management plan relating to prevention, health promotion or rehabilitation was inadequate or inappropriate.
- The plan relating to the medical management of risk was inadequate or inappropriate.
- The implications of co-morbidity were insufficiently considered.
- Uncertainty, including that experienced by the patient, was ineffectively managed.
- Inappropriate or inadequate arrangements for follow-up, continuity and/or safety netting.
- Time management in the consultation was ineffective.

Relating to others:
- Communication skills, verbal and/or non-verbal, including active listening skills, were insufficiently demonstrated.
- The patient's agenda, health belief and/or preferences were insufficiently explored.
- The circumstances, relevant cultural differences and/or preferences of those involved were insufficiently responded to.
- Explanations were inadequately shared or adapted to the person's needs.
- A judgemental approach was shown to the person.
- Respect and/or sensitivity shown to the person was inadequate or inappropriate.
- Ownership of responsibility for decision-making was inadequate or inappropriate.
- Teamwork and/or understanding of others' roles were insufficiently recognised or responded to.
- Safeguarding concerns were inadequately recognised or responded to.

At first sight, this looks to be a forbidding list of pitfalls, and you might wonder how on earth anyone ever passes the SCA, given the number of shortcomings you have to try not to display. But relax – perfection is not necessary to pass, and to pass with flying colours. Indeed, there's no such thing as a perfect consultation. All doctors, examiners included, have good days and bad days, consultations that go well and others where we feel we've let ourselves down. The best anyone can hope for is a consultation that identifies and addresses the patient's problem, results in an outcome that satisfies both patient and doctor, and is conducted smoothly, efficiently, respectfully, and with kindness. These feedback statements are intended primarily as gentle guidance as to aspects of consulting where improvement or development would be beneficial. And this applies to successful candidates as well as unsuccessful ones. It takes more than the odd one or two negative comments to drop the score on an SCA case below the passing standard. For this to happen, the cumulative effect of the errors would have to be sufficient for the patient's safety, dignity or autonomy to be significantly compromised.

So read between the lines of the SCA's standard descriptors and feedback statements, and allow a picture of a safe, independent newly-qualified GP to form in your imagination. Compare yourself to this ideal. It's my guess that, on a good day and in many of your consultations, you're there already, or pretty close. And in that spirit of optimism, read on to Section 4 of this book and see whether any of my hints for making a success of the three-part consultation might be useful.

About the author, illustrator and foreword writers

About the author

Roger Neighbour OBE MA MB BChir DSc FRCP FRCGP FRACGP

Roger qualified from King's College, Cambridge, and St Thomas' Hospital, London. After vocational training in Watford, he practised as a GP in Abbot's Langley, Hertfordshire, from 1974 to 2003. He was a trainer and programme director with the Watford Vocational Training Scheme for many years, an MRCGP examiner for 20 years and the Royal College of General Practitioners' Chief Examiner from 1997 to 2002. In 2003, he was elected President of the RCGP for a three-year term. In 2011, he was made an OBE for services to medical education. Having studied experimental psychology instead of biochemistry as an undergraduate, Roger found himself fascinated by the psychology of the consultation and the doctor–patient relationship in general practice. This interest led him to write his 'Inner' trilogy: *The Inner Consultation* (1987), *The Inner Apprentice* (1992) and *The Inner Physician* (2016). A collection of his medico-philosophical writings, *I'm Too Hot Now*, was published in 2005. Now retired from clinical practice, Roger has continued to write, teach and lecture in the United Kingdom and worldwide on consulting skills and medical education. He is a Visiting Professor of Medical Education at Brunel University Medical School, London. Roger is a practising Zen Buddhist; he plays the violin to semi-professional standard, and is something of an authority on the music of Franz Schubert.

About the illustrator

Jamie Hynes MB ChB FRCGP DRCOG PGCertMedEd

Jamie is an enthusiastic and fulfilled GP, committed husband, and a father to two boys. Qualified from Birmingham in 2002, he is currently a training programme director for West Birmingham VTS and Chair of the RCGP Midland Faculty. He recalls that when, as a medical student, he was questioned about his CV's mention of artistic interests, he described the practice of medicine as an art. He is delighted to keep utilising the creativity from life before training in this book, as well as in his practice, VTS websites and social media activities as @ArtfulDoctor. Jamie's video-poem extolling the virtues and privileges of general practice, 'The National Health,' won the RCGP Midland Faculty's 'Inspiration' competition. Further pieces on general practice followed, with #GP150w (GP in 150 words), and cross-Faculty collaborations such as the Christmas-themed 'The Night Before CQC,' #12daysofGP, and #GPKipling, a video communicating the diversity of our workforce in a GP-themed rewrite of Kipling's 'If.' The #GPKipling video launched the RCGP Annual Conference in 2019, and the Billy Joel–inspired, GP-themed 'Start the Fire' launched the RCGP Annual Conference in 2021. He was awarded RCGP Faculty Champion in 2022. His short illustrated film examining the evidence for continuity of care within a storytelling narrative entitled 'GP's a Wonderful Life' featured on The General Practice Podcast in 2023. His illustrations have featured at an RCGP Annual Conference, in GPfrontline, RCGP InnovAiT and, of course, in Roger Neighbour's *The Inner Physician* (2016).

About the first edition's foreword writer

Helen Stokes-Lampard DBE MBBS(Lon) PhD FRCGP DSc(Med) DFSRH DRCOG

Helen Stokes-Lampard is a practising GP partner in Lichfield, Staffordshire. She was Chair of the Academy of Medical Royal Colleges, the umbrella organisation for all medical disciplines, from 2020 to 2023. She is also a past Chair of the RCGP 2016–2019, having held many other roles there over the years. Additionally, she is a Professor of GP Education at the University of Birmingham and Chair of the National Academy for Social Prescribing, an independent charity established to promote the concepts and build the evidence base around social prescribing. Helen is naturally enthusiastic, a passionate advocate for person-centred care in its widest sense, and an experienced public speaker.

About the second edition's foreword writer

Rich Withnall KHS OStJ MA MD MSc MBBS FRCGP FRCP FAcadMEd SFFMLM CMgr

Rich Withnall is Professor of General Practice, the Royal College of General Practitioners' Chief Examiner, and Medical Director for International Education and Training. He is also Chief Executive and Responsible Officer of the Faculty of Medical Leadership and Management, the professional home for medical leadership in the UK. He qualified from the Royal Free Hospital School of Medicine, University of London, in 1992. He served in the Royal Air Force for 34 years, rising to the rank of Air Vice-Marshal and becoming Director of Defence Healthcare. He has been an Honorary Surgeon to Her Late Majesty Queen Elizabeth II and His Majesty King Charles III.

Acknowledgements

One of the most felicitous meetings of my life was with the Danish GP Dr Jan-Helge Larsen, who for decades has run residential consultation courses on the idyllic Greek island of Kalymnos. Jan-Helge likes my stuff, and I discovered when I first tutored on one of his courses how much I like his. From him, I learned how a core of structure makes a consultation strong enough to carry the weight of knowledge, skill, insight and kindness that doctors aspire to offer their patients. Thank you, Jan.

Jamie Hynes is one of the most positive and committed GPs I know, and is infuriatingly talented. I'm lost in admiration for his ability to make a few lines on paper and have whole stories come to life. Sincere thanks for the artwork and the cover, Jamie – great stuff.

Much of the material in this book was developed for, and tried out on, the CSA preparation courses run by Brigadier (Retd) Robin Simpson for the Midland Faculty of the RCGP. If the book has any relevance or usefulness, it is in no small measure thanks to Robin's long experience with the MRCGP exam and his dedication to helping young doctors to pass it.

I hope Helen Stokes-Lampard realises that inviting her to write the Foreword to the first edition when she's already extraordinarily busy was my way of saying a big 'Thank you for everything you do for general practice.' I'm so glad, Helen, that you said 'Yes.'

Rich Withnall, who has written the Foreword to the second edition, is a wonderful friend and supporter. His gentle modesty belies his clarity of thought and his determination, as the RCGP's Chief Examiner, to see that the MRCGP is the best and fairest of all the career-pivoting exams in the medical firmament. As well as his Foreword, Rich's comments, suggestions and corrections have been invaluable, and I couldn't be more grateful.

Working with Jo Koster and her colleagues at CRC Press/Taylor & Francis is always a pleasure. Every author treats a new book like a newborn child, and it has been enormously reassuring to know that this one is in such safe hands. Thank you, all of you.

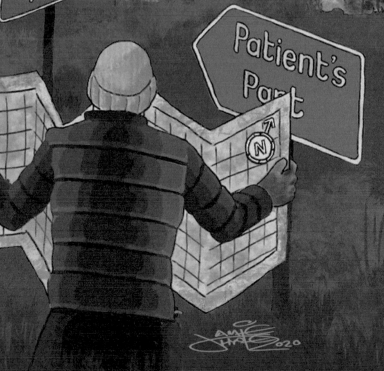

1

As we begin

This book's sub-title is *A practical guide to successful general practice consultations before, during and beyond the MRCGP*, which is quite a mouthful. But every word is important. Let me explain why, starting with …

… 'the MRCGP'

Since 2007, it has been a requirement that, before you can practise unsupervised as a general practitioner (GP) in the United Kingdom, you have to pass the Membership of the Royal College of General Practitioners (MRCGP) exam as part of obtaining a Certificate of Completion of Training. As I expect you know, the MRCGP has three components:

- the Workplace-Based Assessment (WPBA), confirming that you have acquired the necessary range of professional competencies, including physical examination;
- the Applied Knowledge Test (AKT), which is a computer-based assessment of knowledge and problem-solving;
- the Simulated Consultation Assessment (SCA), where you have a series of 12 online video and audio consultations with simulated patients, each lasting 12 minutes, testing your ability to combine your clinical and communication skills into an effective consultation.

The SCA is probably the scariest part. Your interactions with real live persons are going to be watched and judged by a real live examiner. To pass the SCA, it's not enough just to know your medicine; you have to sort out the patient's problem effectively and sensitively, all within

DOI: 10.1201/9781032619200-1

12 minutes – exactly 720 seconds. To do this, you need consulting skills, and you need to use them skilfully to manage the consultation to good effect. If you haven't passed the SCA yet, my aim in this book is to help you acquire these skills and put them into practice.

... 'consultations' ...

'The consultation is at the heart of general practice.' How often have you heard that? Trainers, academics and practising GPs all agree that there are skills in managing the *process* of the consultation – the *how you do it* – which are different from, and additional to, the clinical skills needed to deal with its medical *content* – the *what you do*. But does this matter? After all, a consultation is really only a conversation, you talking to a patient. And how hard can *that* be? You have perfectly satisfactory conversations every day of your life. True – but a medical consultation is a conversation *with a point*. Or two points, actually. For the patient, the point is to get some help with what they think is a medical problem. For you the doctor, the point is to gain the satisfaction of a job well done (and to earn your living) by putting to good use the professional knowledge you have spent years acquiring. And once a conversation has a point, a purpose, there is a responsibility to do whatever it takes to achieve that purpose. And because we doctors are the professionals, the ones with the expertise, that responsibility is mainly ours. The onus is on us to see that, within the limits of what's possible and realistic, the patients get what they need from the consultation.

... 'general practice' ...

Seen through the eyes of hospital medicine, general practice can look like a foreign country; we do things differently here.

By the time patients reach a hospital ward or clinic, they have usually been filtered and preselected. To make sure they are in the right department, their problems have already been, or quickly are, categorised according either to the organ system affected (e.g. orthopaedics, ophthalmology) or to the nature of the disease (e.g. oncology, psychiatry). A consultation between a patient and a hospital doctor typically follows the sequence we were all taught at medical school: history, examination and investigations, leading to diagnosis and then on to treatment. At medical school and during our early years in hospital medicine, this familiar structure becomes so deeply ingrained that we tend to believe it is the best and only way of working. And indeed, it can be very effective – as long as the patient's disease is relatively clear-cut and their individual idiosyncrasies don't matter too much.

But as you know, in general practice, the problems our patients bring are not always well defined or readily classified. Any physical pathology they might have is affected by psychological, emotional, social, cultural and economic influences. The patient's personal background, circumstances, beliefs and preferences all have to be factored into our assessment and management. And as if this wasn't complicated enough, there is the added pressure in the United Kingdom of having only 10 minutes, on average, to do it in.

... 'successful' ...

In the context of this seemingly impossible task, what makes a general practice consultation a 'successful' one? Ideally, at the end of 10 minutes or so, the patient would leave your consulting room feeling better, or relieved, or better informed, or at least knowing they are in safe hands. You, for your part, want to be left feeling quietly satisfied, thinking *That went well*, knowing that you had practised good medicine and at the same time had been helpful to a fellow human being. In the real world, of course, this 'two happy people' outcome is not always achievable. There will often be a degree of compromise, or disappointment, or frustration, or doubt, or of 'more needs to be done.' One party – doctor or patient – may end up being more satisfied than the other. But the important thing is to rate the success of the consultation not just by purely medical criteria but also by whether the patient feels they have benefitted from it.

If the consultation in question is an SCA case, 'successful' would mean scoring maximum marks in every section of the marking schedule: 'data gathering and diagnosis,' 'clinical management and medical complexity' and 'relating to others.' Here too, however, successful does not have to mean perfect. To score full marks, it's enough to do only as much as a decent GP could reasonably be expected to do under the circumstances and in the time available.

... 'during' ...

All exams are stressful, and the SCA is particularly so. In an exam, when you're nervous and full of adrenalin, it's easy to forget the principles of good consulting you've learned during your training. You'll worry that you won't perform as well as you do back home in your practice. Inevitably, during the three hours or so that the SCA lasts, some cases will go better than others. There will be times when you think you're on completely the wrong lines and are missing the point. There may be times when you feel that you and the patient are at cross purposes or your mind just goes blank. You want your consultations to have some structure, so that you can be competent and thorough, yet at the same time patient-centred and caring. But you don't want the structure to be so rigid and obvious that you come across as a robot. Doing all this under exam conditions is really hard.

Luckily, the examiners, who themselves are all working GPs, know and understand the pressure you are under. And despite what you might imagine, they are *not* out to trap you or make you jump through arbitrary hoops. Nevertheless, they do need to see that you can deliver the safe and effective care your future patients have the right to expect. And they can only base their judgement on what you can show them during the exam.

To help you do your best on the day, to cover the essential points in 12 minutes, to give you a sense of security in your consulting skills that will keep your nerves under control, and to give you a kind of 'lifebelt' to rescue you if things start to go wrong, you need a framework for your consultations. I think you need a framework that:

- is **simple** – i.e. easy to understand, learn and remember;
- **makes sense** – i.e. feels right and natural, and is clearly rooted in the real world of general practice;
- is **comprehensive** – i.e. fits a wide range of problems and situations;
- is **adaptable** – i.e. works in unfamiliar or unexpected situations;
- is **robust under pressure** – i.e. easy to recall if you get flustered, and helps you get back on track if things go wrong;
- is **SCA-friendly** – i.e. helps you do as well under exam conditions as you know you can do on a good day back in your usual workplace;
- **gets you into good habits** – i.e. lays the basis for a consulting style that will stand you in good stead throughout your career after you've passed the MRCGP; and
- quickly **becomes second nature** – so that a general practice consulting style becomes your default way of consulting, even under pressure.

It's for you, of course, to judge whether the approach I describe in this book delivers on these ambitions. But I hope and believe it goes at least some way towards meeting them.

EXAM POINT: Finding out about the SCA

For accurate and up-to-date information about the SCA's regulations, arrangements, dates, etc., there is only one completely reliable source – the RCGP website https://www.rcgp.org.uk/mrcgp-exams/simulated-consultation-assessment. Do not rely on any other websites, articles, courses or books that are not produced by the RCGP or its Faculties – not even this one! The staff of the College's Examination Department will also be unfailingly helpful. Their contact details are on the website.

... 'before' ...

I'd really like you to be reading this book long before you sit the SCA, preferably early in your GP training; even, maybe, as a medical student or Foundation Year doctor. Why?

There's a Zen story of a young monk who went to his Master and asked, 'Master, how should I lead a perfect life?' The Master replied, 'First, make yourself perfect. Then – live naturally' (Figure 1.1).

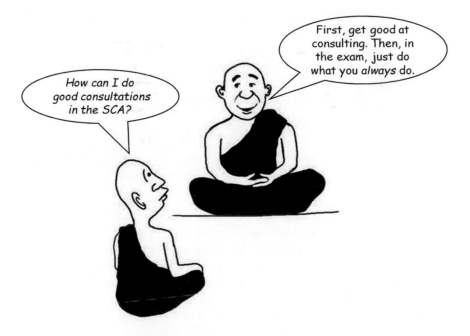

FIGURE 1.1

The lesson is, don't leave it until the last moment before you try to get your consulting up to exam standards. Get interested in the art and skill of consulting early in your GP training. It takes a while to upgrade your old hospital-style consultations to the more patient-centred approach needed in general practice. Practise GP-style consulting – with the help of your trainer, your colleagues and books like this – until you're doing it without having to think about it. Then, on the day of the exam, just go in and do what you always do.

Don't approach the SCA as if you were auditioning for a part in a film. One of the saddest things an examiner sees is a candidate putting on what is obviously a performance, play-acting the role of what they think is the kind of doctor the RCGP wants to see. The examiners can easily tell the phoney from the genuine. Expressions of interest or sympathy that don't ring true; badly timed or formulaic enquiries about ideas, concerns and expectations; clumsy attempts at shared decision-making that come across as patronising – they all make the candidate sound like an under-rehearsed actor and are tell-tale signs that the general practice way of consulting is not yet securely embedded. It's better to start your preparation much earlier, so that, come the exam, what you show the examiners is a true reflection of what, by then, has become your usual way of talking to patients.

But what if you've left it late and have only a few weeks, even days, before you sit the SCA? Don't despair. You can very quickly pick up two or three key ideas and suggestions from this book and try them out over the course of a week in your everyday practice. Even this will have a beneficial and confidence-boosting effect. You will find some practical suggestions in the chapter on 'Some particular challenges.'

... 'and beyond' ...

If the SCA is still ahead of you, passing it is probably enough of a goal to motivate you to work on your consulting skills. But after you have passed the MRCGP – what then? A share or salaried partnership? A portfolio career? Locums? Working abroad? Wherever your career takes you, assuming you continue to see patients, you will spend much of your time conducting consultations. What will happen to the consulting skills you so diligently acquired as a trainee? We know from research carried out in the RCGP in the 1990s that an individual's consulting style takes some time to reach its final form; you will continue to develop your own style for several years after you finish your formal GP training.

Once your training is complete, general practice exposes you to fresh pressures. There is never enough time; patients' expectations seem to grow inexorably, and some of them seem unrealistic or downright unreasonable; and you will have to shoulder your share of administrative and managerial tasks as well. In the face of these challenges, it is all too easy to revert to a brusquer, more doctor-centred style of consulting. What is more, you will no longer have a trainer on hand to offer you advice, support and encouragement. The consulting room can be a lonely place; there is no one there to notice if you start to slip into bad habits without realising it.

For some of your peers, the stresses of real-life practice will gnaw away at their interpersonal skills until every consultation becomes a battle for supremacy between doctor and patient. But for others – and I hope you are amongst them – seeing patients and having good consultations will remain a career-long source of satisfaction and fulfilment. Knowing that your consulting skills are equal to any challenge is the best antidote to burnout. And equipping you with challenge-resistant consulting skills is the aim of this book.

... 'practical guide' ...

It ought to go without saying that there is no single 'right' way of consulting. (I say 'ought' because you sometimes hear it said that there is an official RCGP model of the consultation that you have to stick to in the SCA. This is a myth.) But there certainly *are* ways of consulting that help you deliver good patient-centred care that are time-efficient and satisfying to both you and your patient.

I want this book to help you establish ways of thinking, talking and behaving in the consultation that are most likely to lead to a good outcome. Note that word *outcome*. Outcome is more important than process. What you achieve in the consultation is more important than how you do it. It is more important that your consultations achieve their aim than that you get too hung up on the techniques you might employ, such as open questions or summarising.

That said, there is a natural sequence to an effective consultation, and it's not complicated. Think of the consultation as falling into three consecutive parts (Figure 1.2):

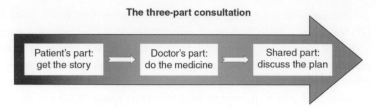

The three-part consultation

Start by getting the patient's account of the problem as fully as possible.

Then get whatever additional information you need in order to understand it in medical terms.

Then discuss and negotiate a plan of action until you're both happy.

FIGURE 1.2

1 the **Patient's part**, in which you encourage the patient to tell you everything they want or need to say about their problem, in their own way.

2 the **Doctor's part**, when you gather whatever additional information you need to make a professional medical assessment of the problem.

3 the **Shared part**, where you and the patient together work your way to a management plan that you both feel satisfied with.

The next section of this book, *The big picture*, is a preamble setting its main ideas in context. If you're not interested in why you might benefit from this approach, or in knowing its underlying principles, or how it fits in with other ideas about the consultation – then don't bother reading it. But I hope you will.

Then come two sections – *The consultation in a nutshell* and *Making a success of the three-part consultation* – which go into all the detail. They explain and expand on this three-part sequence and show you how you can make it happen smoothly and efficiently. But please don't take it as a 'one-size-fits-all' recipe for success. As you read, imagine that you and I are having a series of tutorials, where I make some suggestions and you think about whether they are sensible or helpful.

After this comes a section dealing with some of the challenges and difficulties which, I know from experience, are of particular concern to those of you preparing for the SCA, but which also crop up in everyday general practice. You will also find some advice on how best to prepare for the exam.

Finally, there's a postscript called *Before you go.* Passing the MRCGP is not an end in itself. I hope that, with the exam no longer hanging over your head, you will want your consulting style to continue to evolve and mature, so that your ability to create sometimes life-pivoting interactions with your patients remains a source of quiet pride for the rest of your career.

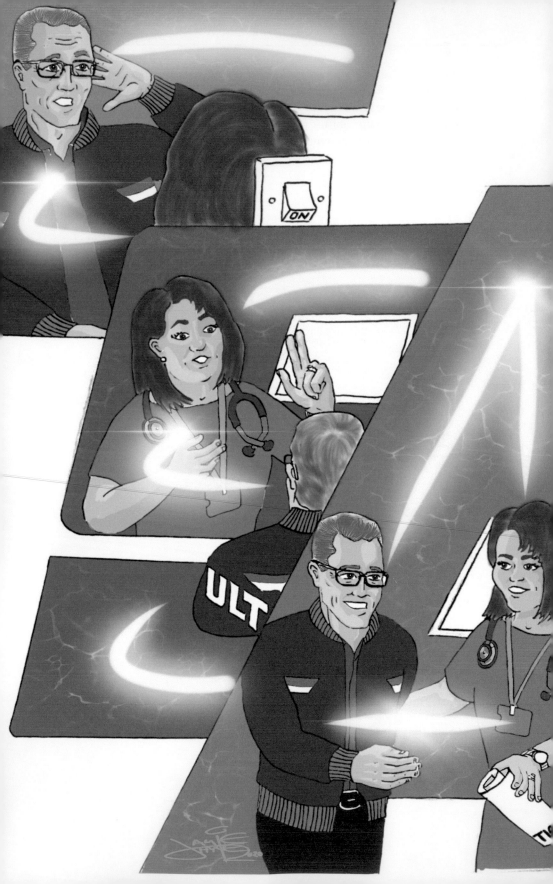

2

The big picture

I don't know about you, but when I'm trying to take new ideas on board, I like to have a sense of the big picture before I get down to the detail. I want to know that there is some point to them; that it is worth making the effort to understand them; and that any new information fits in with, builds on, or possibly challenges what I think I know already. If I'm reading a book, I want to feel reasonably confident that I'll be able to make it through to the end and that I'll benefit in some way if I do. So in this preamble, I am unashamedly trying to soften you up to be receptive to the ideas about 'the consultation in a nutshell' which I'll be telling you about in later sections of the book. (If, on the other hand, you prefer to start with the core detail and then work outwards, you could skip this section for now and come back to it later.)

If you *are* reading this preamble, a word of caution! Don't expect it necessarily to form a single, unwavering line of argument, unfolding in a clear, linear fashion from start to finish. In this book, I am trying to transmit an interconnected set of ideas from my mind to yours through the medium of language, one word after another. I have, to the best of my ability, to convert the thoughts in my head into a sequence of words on a page. And then it's over to you. From my stream of words, you have to reconstruct, in *your* head and to the best of *your* ability, what it is you think I am trying to communicate. I don't have any control over how you do that. I can only hope that the mental edifice you build bears some resemblance to the one I have in mind. You may find some of the things that I say in this section interesting and relevant; others perhaps less so. But I don't know which bits you will readily understand, and which bits will pass you by. So, all I can do is a kind of 'data dump.' I'll offload the various ideas that are in the front of my mind at this point in my narrative and leave it to you to piece them together as best you can, hoping that you won't get prematurely seduced by some and prejudiced against others.

In many ways, my situation is like that of the patient who consults you. He (or she) wants to get across to you something that is important but not always easily articulated. He tries to explain, using the only tool at his command – language. He may not find the right words, and he can't be sure that you will interpret what he says in the way that he intends. All he can do is tell you his story *his* way, and hope that you are imaginative enough and empathic enough to understand.

The message is the same to you, the doctor, as to you, the reader: don't rush to judgement. Don't be too quick to accept or reject every phrase, every sentence, every paragraph. Allow what you hear or read to wash over you, letting yourself resonate with it as your past experience dictates. Give it time to sink in. Don't worry if you can't immediately see the point of what is being said to you. If there *is* significance to be found, let it find itself. If questions and opinions form in your mind, park them for the time being. The time to interrogate and clarify, the time to impose structure and meaning on the narrative, comes soon – but not yet. For now, let me – and in the consultation, your patient – tell it my way – his way – first.

This book's central concept – the consultation's three-part structure – needs a lucid and coherent explanation, and in the next chapter I'll do my best to provide it. But its background, its context, its philosophy and its reason for being cannot be so straightforwardly told. Before I get to the specifics, allow me first to set the scene in my own way. Your reward for doing so is the possibility of an understanding that will make better sense of my main narrative.

Here again, I could be the voice of your patient: *You must allow me first to tell my story in my own way; and your reward for doing so is the possibility of a better understanding of why I've come to see you.*

You'll probably notice that, from time to time, I seem to be repeating something I've said already, although maybe expressing it a bit differently. I don't apologise for this. As an author addressing an unknown reader, I have no way of knowing whether, just because I've said something once, you have understood and absorbed it. Indeed, if you're anything like me, it helps to have important messages reinforced in a variety of ways. Here's the first; let's remind ourselves of the goals of a general practice consultation.

What are the goals of the consultation?

Essentially, the consultation is a process for converting a problem into a plan. That's so important that I'm going to say it again.

The consultation is a process for converting a problem into a plan.

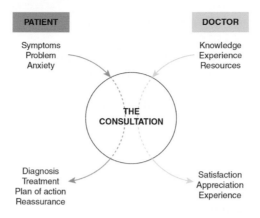

FIGURE 2.1

In a general practice consultation (Figure 2.1), two people – patient and doctor – meet to exchange information, mainly for the benefit of one of them, usually the patient. The patient usually comes with a problem of some kind – symptoms, anxieties or questions – which they think the GP will be able to help with. The doctor brings his or her medical knowledge and experience, plus the ability to access all the technological and organisational resources of the health service. By the end of the consultation, the patient hopes to have at least a partial solution to their problem. This might be a diagnosis, some treatment or a plan of action, advice, reassurance, or information. The doctor hopes to end the consultation satisfied with a job well done, knowing that they have made an appreciable (and, one hopes, appreciated) difference to the patient's health or well-being.

In the British NHS, patients are free to present whatever problem they choose to a GP, which is why the MRCGP curriculum appears so dauntingly large. However, not all of a patient's problems and needs fall within the scope of the doctor's responsibility or competence, and any given problem does not require the doctor to draw upon all the resources available. For example, it is your duty to help a patient's arthritis, but not his bank overdraft or his dislike of his mother-in-law. Conversely, faced with a patient who has what is clearly tennis elbow, you are not obliged to arrange an MRI scan or a specialist referral, even though these options are theoretically open to you. Some problems, such as marital or sexual difficulties and some minor mental health issues, are matters for negotiation as to whether they fall within a GP's remit. Similarly, individual GPs differ as to whether or not they offer particular skills such as counselling, minor surgery or family planning. So another goal of the consultation is, where necessary, to negotiate the area of overlap between what the patient wants and what the doctor can provide.

Converting a problem into a plan

Every time you see a patient – every time *any* doctor sees *any* patient – the consultation goes through the same two stages:

• First, you work out what the problem is that needs your attention.
• Then, you work out what is to be done about it.

Of course, it takes tremendous professional knowledge and training to do this effectively. You have to know a lot of medicine, be good at diagnosis, have a sound knowledge of therapeutics, have good judgement and empathy, be a good communicator and so on. But essentially, in process terms, what doctors do is not much different from what a car mechanic does – identify the problem, then come up with a plan to try and sort it.

The important thing about this simple strategy is the order of events. Finding out the problem comes *before* deciding what to do about it. We shouldn't commit to a plan of action until we are sure that it is addressing the *right* problem. And the 'right' problem – the one we need to focus on – isn't always the obvious one, or the first one we come across, or the one that is most convenient. Sometimes, if we are stressed or inexperienced, we are tempted to reverse the order and make the problem suit the plan we have already decided on. We have all been guilty of such thoughts as, *If it's dermatology, I'll try some steroid cream*, or *It can't be cardiac pain, it's nearly six o'clock*. It's also important not to sign off on a plan of action until both parties – you and your patient – are happy with it and agree that it is the right thing to do.

Although this two-stage account of the consultation process is very simple, it is nonetheless valid in even the most complicated consultations. Indeed, when things are complicated or you get flustered, it is even more important to 'see the wood for the trees' and remember: be clear about what the real problem is, and only then move on to planning a course of action. And it's particularly important in an SCA case. The question that should be in your mind, guiding everything you say and do at the beginning of the consultation, should be *What's the real problem here? What are we going to do about it?* comes later.

Whose version of 'the problem'?

In order to work out what a patient's real problem is, you need data – information. Obviously, your primary source of data is the patient. Information comes from the story the patient tells you, in words and non-verbal communication, and also from the story told by their body in the form of physical signs. The trouble is, the stories patients tell at the start of their consultations are often a mix of high-grade and low-grade information, and sometimes no information at all.

Let's imagine a patient who begins the consultation by saying, 'This is my wife's idea ... Anyway, I've been getting a bit of gyp in the old tummy, and the number twos have gone a bit, I don't know what you'd call it, iffy. I expect you'll tell me it's nothing.'

A story like this is hard to 'do medicine' on. During your medical training, you weren't taught the causes of 'gyp,' or the anatomical structure of the 'tummy,' or how to investigate 'iffy-ness of the number twos.' And you can't be sure how to interpret remarks like, *This is my wife's idea* or *I expect you'll tell me it's nothing*. The patient's account of the problem seems to make sense to him, and it gives you a starting point, but it is ambiguous, vague and incomplete. You have, somehow, to translate the patient's story into a version more suitable for doctors, such as: *The patient has a four-week history of intermittent low abdominal pain and change of bowel habit. He and his wife are worried it could be cancer.*

Now you have the beginnings of a version of the problem you can do general practice medicine on. Having now translated the patient's narrative into medical terms, your medical training prompts you to fill in the missing details, ask your 'red flag' questions about blood in the stools and weight loss, enquire about relevant risk factors, and explore the thoughts and fears of the patient and his wife. Then you will have achieved what I like to call 'insight on the verge of action'; you will be in a position to make a comprehensive assessment of the patient's problem and ready to move on from 'problem identification' to 'action planning.'

But you have only reached this position of in-depth understanding by first attending to the patient's story in an open-minded way, not only sifting it for medical information but also picking up the nuances in the way it was told. This is why, in the approach to the consultation this book describes, the patient gets to go first. The patient gets to tell their story in their own way, on their own terms, *before* the doctor sets about massaging it into a form more amenable to medical analysis and intervention.

What good consulting is, and is not

Good consulting is *not* ...

- ... like performing in a circus, where you get to show off your lion-taming skills by subduing a fierce and predatory creature (the patient) through sheer strength of will. Nor is it like juggling, where you have to keep an increasing number of balls in the air without dropping any.

- It's not about parading your repertoire of stock phrases and gimmicky communication skills like a car salesman.
- It's not about trying to manipulate the patient into agreeing with you or doing what you want them to.
- Neither is it about letting the patient dictate the agenda and make all the decisions.
- Consulting in general practice is not doing hospital medicine, only faster.
- It's not a counsel of perfection, unachievable in real life.
- And it's not about slavishly following anyone's theoretical model of the consultation – not even mine.

Good consulting *is* …

- … bringing all your professional skills – clinical and communicational – to bear on the individual patient's problem.
- It's having a consultation structure and using a consultation process that allow you to help the patient to the best of your ability in the time available.
- It's about being able to tell what matters to the patient, and about getting from the patient the information that matters to *you*.
- It's about knowing what needs to happen in order for both you and the patient to be happy with the outcome.
- And it's about knowing how to *make* it happen, in the time available, moving the consultation on and keeping it on track if necessary.
- When it comes to decision-making, it's about treating the patient as your colleague, not your master or your slave, or your enemy, or your customer.
- Not least, good consulting – consulting in ways that you can be proud of – is what, in the long run, will keep you enjoying your career in general practice.

What consultation models are, and are not

You can't get very far into specialist training for general practice, at least in the UK, without someone telling you about consultation models. A model – a theoretical structure and agenda – seems to have become to the consultation what an indoor toilet was to post-war housing – an 'of-*course*-I've-got-one, how–did–we–ever–manage–without–them' necessity for civilised existence.

The 1980s and 1990s were the heydays of consultation modelling, seeing the publication of what are still probably the 'big four':

- Stott and Davis[1]
- Pendleton[2]
- The Inner Consultation[3]
- Calgary–Cambridge[4]

There is still much to be gained from reading and studying the analysis and advice of these authors, even though they were all writing before the CSA or SCA existed and at a time when general practice was arguably less pressured than it currently is. One unintended consequence of this body of literature, however, has been the erroneous belief that, to pass the SCA, you have to use the right consultation model and stick to it rigidly. This is a myth. There *is* no 'right' RCGP-approved model of the consultation, not in the SCA or anywhere else. The myth stems partly from the fact that the word 'model' has several different meanings and nuances, not all of which feel appropriate in the context of the consulting room.

According to the Oxford English Dictionary, a model is:

1   a simplified description of a system or process to assist calculations and predictions;

2   a representation of a person, thing or proposed structure, typically on a smaller scale than the original;

3   a person or thing regarded as an excellent example of a specified quality.

---

[1] Stott NCH and Davis RH. (1979). The exceptional potential in each primary care consultation. J R Coll Gen Pract. 29:201–205. Four possible things to do: deal with the presenting problem; manage continuing problems; opportunistic health promotion; and modify help-seeking behaviour.

[2] Pendleton D, Schofield T, Tate P and Havelock P. (1984). *The Consultation: An Approach to Learning and Teaching.* Oxford: Oxford University Press. Seven consultation tasks: define the reason for the patient's attendance; consider other problems; choose appropriate action(s); achieve shared understanding; involve the patient in management; use time and resources appropriately; and establish or maintain doctor–patient relationship. This is the origin of the ICE (Ideas, Concerns and Expectations) mnemonic.

[3] Neighbour R. (1987, 2nd ed. 2005). The Inner Consultation: *How to Develop an Effective and Intuitive Consulting Style.* Abingdon: Taylor & Francis. Five 'checkpoints' to be reached in turn: connecting, summarising, hand-over, safety-netting and housekeeping.

[4] Kurtz SM, Silverman JD and Draper J. (1998). Teaching and Learning Communication Skills in Medicine. Oxford: Radcliffe Medical Press. Better known as the Calgary-Cambridge guide to the medical interview. A framework with five elements: initiating the session; gathering information; building the relationship; explanation and planning; and closing the session. Describes (at the last count) 71 separate component skills.

When we speak of a 'model' citizen, we mean someone who conforms to society's norms so completely that the powers-that-be wish everybody would do the same. A 'model' child is exemplary in looks and behaviour, obedient to adult expectations and causing no trouble. To 'model' clothes is to show off someone else's creations to best advantage; and the 'models' who do so are generally admired more for their surface appearance than for their depth or individuality.

'Model' in the sense of a model aeroplane comes close to what we mean by a consultation model – a simplified representation of the key features of an object or process as an aid to understanding. But even here, there are ambiguities. Look at the three models of an airliner in Figure 2.2. Which is the best? You can't say; it depends on what key features you are interested in. If you just want to recognise a Boeing 747 when you see one, model 1 is probably the most useful. If you want the exact measurements of its component parts, model 2 provides that information. If you want to understand how its engines generate thrust, model 3 will give you the best idea.

So what is a consultation model *for*? It's not a set of rules for how to conduct your interactions with patients. It's not a recipe guaranteeing a good outcome. It's not a description of perfection. It's not a shortcut to exam

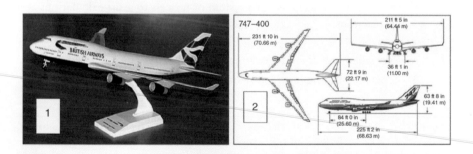

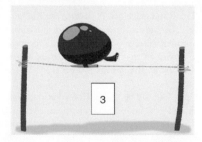

Which is the best model of a Boeing 747?

FIGURE 2.2

success. It's not, as is occasionally suggested, part of an establishment plot to clone GPs into some predetermined mould. It's a teaching aid.

Think of it this way. Suppose you were invited into the cockpit of an airliner and saw the Captain smoothly flying the plane with seemingly effortless skill. A slight pressure on the yoke, the occasional flick of a switch, a few unfamiliar words spoken into a headset, and the miracle of flight unfolds. 'How are you doing that?' you ask. 'Ah,' comes the knowing reply, 'training, experience and flair. Man and machine in harmony.' *That's too vague, it doesn't explain anything*, you think. You persist; 'No, really, I want to understand what's going through your head, because I might like to train as a pilot myself one day.' So the Captain explains. 'Rule number one: Aviate, Navigate, Communicate. Four forces on the aircraft – gravity, lift, thrust and drag. The airways are like motorways in three dimensions …' What the Captain is giving you is a model – his attempt to transfer into *your* mind something of what is in *his* mind when he is carrying out the skills you yourself might like to acquire. Another Captain, when asked the same question, might give you a 'surgeon-in-an-operating-theatre' model, or a 'concert-pianist-performing-a-concerto' model. All would add something to your understanding of how pilots go about their work, but the added 'something' would be different in each case. You might find one model more helpful than another, but none of them could or would claim to be the 'right' one. If, in due course, you did indeed take flying lessons, you would probably find that the ideas that had been represented to you through the Captains' models contributed to a framework around which you could organise your understanding. But it would be your *own* understanding, not an exact facsimile of any of theirs.

So a consultation model is just a way of trying to speed up the transfer of expertise from a doctor with some skill in consulting to someone else still in the learning stages.

Something else, consultation models are not

They are not assessment tools for measuring or evaluating the quality of your consultations.

A consultation model is not a checklist of things you should try to do in every consultation. No one should attempt to give you marks for how closely you adhere to any particular model. Still less should you think in terms of 'passing' or 'failing' in your use of models. You can be sure that the SCA examiners don't think this way.

The moral is, have a framework for your consultations, but don't try to stick to it slavishly. Tailor your approach to the needs of the individual

1. DATA-GATHERING, TECHNICAL AND ASSESSMENT SKILLS:
   Gathering & using data for clinical judgement, choice of examination, investigations & their interpretation.
   Demonstrating proficiency in performing physical examinations & using diagnostic and therapeutic instruments.

2. CLINICAL MANAGEMENT SKILLS:
   Recognition & management of common medical conditions in primary care.
   Demonstrating a structured & flexible approach to decision-making.
   Demonstrating the ability to deal with multiple complaints and co-morbidity.
   Demonstrating the ability to promote a positive approach to health.

3. INTERPERSONAL SKILLS:
   Demonstrating the use of recognised communication techniques to gain understanding of the patient's illness experience and develop a shared approach to managing problems.
   Practicising ethically with respect for equality and diversity issues, in line with the accepted codes of professional conduct.

The 3 CSA assessment domains

FIGURE 2.3

patient in front of you. The purpose of having some structure is so that you can give your best to your patient, not so that an imaginary examiner can tick non-existent boxes on a hypothetical checklist.

The SCA examiners don't work from a checklist or tick boxes to mark whether you do or don't say or do particular things. They don't endorse any particular consultation model; and they don't mind what model you use, or even whether you have one at all, as long as your consultations are effective. They're more interested in what you achieve than in how you do it.

The examiner will be marking your performance in each of three 'assessment domains' (Figure 2.3):

• Data gathering and diagnosis
• Clinical management and medical complexity
• Relating to others

For each case, in each of the three domains, your performance will be rated '*Clear pass*' (scoring 3 marks), '*Pass*' (2 marks), '*Fail*' (1 mark) or '*Clear fail*' (0 marks), making a maximum possible score of 9 marks. In addition to this basic marking schedule, the examiners will have some 'positive or negative indicators' – case-specific pointers suggesting good or less good performance – to help them decide how many marks to award. But note that nowhere in the marking schedule is there any explicit mention of a consultation model. To be sure, there are clear indications that your consulting style is important: *'Adopting a structured approach to problem-solving,' 'using various consulting approaches'* and *'reaching a shared understanding with the patient'*. But these are ideas common to all the standard consultation models. So what matters is not which model you use, but rather the use you make of it to create an effective consultation in the 12 minutes available.

How does the 'three-part' framework fit in with other consultation models?

Now that you understand that the various consultation models are all maps of the same territory, you will see that there is no fundamental conflict between them. They have no ultimate 'truth' beyond their usefulness. They all agree on the outcome they are trying to bring about, i.e., a competent piece of medicine that satisfies the patient's needs. They all broadly agree, also, about the means of achieving this outcome. You need to gain an in-depth understanding of what it is that the patient wants or needs. You need to gather sufficient information, both clinical and contextual, to understand the nature and causes of the patient's problem. You need a comprehensive and up-to-date knowledge of clinical medicine. You need to be able to develop a management plan that is acceptable to the patient as well as to yourself. And you need interpersonal and communication skills to make the consultation run smoothly and sustain the doctor–patient relationship in the long term.

Although I have not yet explained the three-part framework in detail, it is summarised in Figure 2.4. I hope you will see that, in principle, it sits comfortably within this tradition.

The differences between the standard consultation models are more linguistic than conceptual. Different authors use different language to describe what are essentially similar ideas. Many trainers have a preference for one

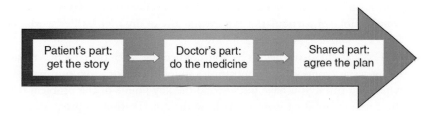

FIGURE 2.4

particular model, finding that it chimes best with their preferred way of teaching. The same is true of many trainees, who find one model suits their learning style better than others. Underlying all the models, however, is the consensus view that, to achieve an effective consultation, it is not enough to know your medicine and to feel well-intentioned towards your patient; there has to be some structure as well.

One criticism to which all the standard models are vulnerable stems from their history. They were all developed before the SCA or its predecessors came into being, with the requirement that the consultation be complete within exactly 10 minutes. Moreover, they all originate from a perhaps more leisured time in general practice: a time before the internet, a time before the Quality and Outcomes Framework, a time when patients usually brought only a single problem, a time when it didn't matter too much if your surgeries overran. None of the standard models, my own Inner Consultation included, addresses the issue of how to do a decent job under pressure and in limited time, under exam conditions or in real life.

The three-part model, carried out in the ways I'll explain in this book, does just this. It:

- is simple enough for you to remember even under exam pressure,
- feels natural,
- can be applied in virtually every clinical situation,
- gets the right balance between the patient's and the doctor's priorities,
- accepts that a degree of 'steering' by the doctor is necessary if the consultation is to achieve its goals in a limited time, and
- fits neatly with the SCA's marking procedures.

The idea of three parts to the consultation is not the creation of any single person, and indeed, it has been around for a long time. I first came across it when I worked with my friend, the Danish GP, Dr Jan-Helge Larsen. Jan-Helge has run consultation courses using this approach on the Greek island of Kalymnos, mainly for Scandinavian doctors, for many years. One of its beauties is how well it harmonises with other established literature on consultation. In particular, it is a natural ally of my own earlier work, *The Inner Consultation*, as Figure 2.5 shows.

The 'Patient's part' begins by you 'connecting' with the patient, creating the necessary rapport and opportunity to tell their story. By 'summarising' when you think you have understood the key points of the problem from the patient's point of view, you allow the consultation to progress to the 'Doctor's part,' where you complete your gathering of the information you need in order to assess the situation from a medical perspective. An update

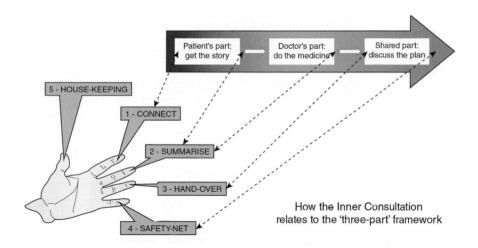

How the Inner Consultation
relates to the 'three-part' framework

FIGURE 2.5

to your summary at the end of the Doctor's part signals the end of data-gathering and the start of the 'Shared action-planning' part. 'Hand-over' suggests that action planning is not complete until the patient is happy with the plan and is ready to take ownership of it. 'Safety-netting' is an important element of the Shared part. *The Inner Consultation*'s final checkpoint, 'housekeeping' – keeping your mind, body and spirits in good order – does not explicitly feature in the three-part model. But housekeeping will be important during the actual SCA exam, when you will need to try to control your nerves, stay fresh and positive for each successive case, and not worry about the ones you have done or those still to come.

Do we really need another model of consultation?

Or another book about it? Or about the SCA? Aren't there enough already?

You'd think so, wouldn't you? Yet despite the abundant literature about the consultation and the large amount of time spent teaching consulting skills, running an effective consultation remains a challenge for significant numbers of GPs at every career stage. Many colleagues in practice, the MRCGP safely behind them, find themselves feeling somewhat helpless in the face of relentlessly rising patient expectations and increasing time pressure. They wonder whether the patient-centred consulting styles they were taught in training are still realistic in today's real-world conditions. And as far as SCA candidates are concerned, although the vast majority will ultimately pass the exam, on average, nearly one candidate in four will fail it at

Examiners' feedback statements (2015-16 CSA diets)	UKGs	Non-UKGs
Management plan under-developed or not reflecting current best practice	13%	19%
Does not recognise issues or priorities in the consultation	9%	14%
Does not develop shared management plan in partnership with patient	6%	12%
Does not use language relevant or understandable to patient	4%	11%
Poor time management	6%	10%
Inappropriate use of resources, including budgetary	7%	10%
Poor awareness and management of risk	8%	10%
Poor active listening skills & use of cues. Consulting formulaic, lacks fluency	3%	10%
Fails to identify abnormal findings or results	6%	9%
Disorganised/unstructured consultation	4%	8%
Does not make correct working or differential diagnosis	6%	8%
Poor rapport, lacks awareness of pt's agenda, health beliefs or preferences	4%	8%
Lacks competence in physical examination	4%	7%
Inadequate safety-netting or follow-up	4%	6%
Does not identify or use psychological or social information	4%	6%
Misses health promotion opportunities	1%	2%

FIGURE 2.6

any given attempt, with weakness in consulting skills largely contributing to their lack of success.

The examiners record their comments on each candidate's performance in the form of 'feedback statements,'[5] and the RCGP periodically publishes an anonymised summary of them. Figure 2.6 is a table showing the commonest reasons for candidates' underperformance; the figures represent the total of all cases that attracted that feedback comment.[6] Figures relating to candidates who are graduates of UK medical schools are shown in the 'UKGs' column, and those for graduates of overseas medical schools in the 'Non-UKGs' column.

In the table, I've used ***bold italic*** emphasis for those comments that reflect on candidates' consulting skills. Moreover, even the commonest criticism, 'underdeveloped management plan,' often stems from the doctor spending so long on data-gathering as to leave insufficient time to move on to the 'management planning' part of the consultation.

---

[5] There are full details of the feedback statements in the *Addendum – Reassurance to SCA candidates* near the start of this book.

[6] Source: Chief Examiner's annual report to the RCGP Council. This data relates to the CSA exams of 2015–2016. At the time of writing, no equivalent analysis is available for the SCA, though it is likely to be broadly similar.

The difference between the exam performance of UK- and non-UK-qualified doctors is not unique to the MRCGP and has been the subject of much debate, analysis and even legal action.[7] The reasons for it are complex, but they are probably largely due to the cultural differences that exist between healthcare systems in various countries.

During their specialist training, aspiring GPs have to make a transition from the doctor-centred approach they learned in medical school and practised in hospitals to the more patient-centred approach that British patients have come to expect in general practice under the NHS. They have to broaden the concept of illness to include its psychological, emotional, social and cultural aspects as well as its purely physical ones. They have to learn to read between the lines and beneath the surface of what patients tell them. And they have to speed up their consulting so that they can bring each consultation to a successful conclusion within roughly 10 minutes. These are difficult tasks, and they are all the harder for international medical graduates. If you have learned your medicine in a country where the doctor is traditionally regarded as a figure of authority, it is a greater cultural shift for you to move to a style of medicine where listening is as important as telling and the patient's point of view has to be actively factored into your decision-making. If your first language is not English, it will be more difficult for you to interpret the nuances in what your patients tell you, and the way you talk to them may not be as fluent as your colleagues who have been speaking colloquial English all their lives.

The three-part model described in this book is my attempt to put effective consulting firmly within the grasp of colleagues who, for whatever reason, find it challenging. It takes a fresh look at the key features of traditional approaches to consulting, simplifies them where possible and updates them to fit more comfortably with present-day constraints of time and resources. I hope it will help you concentrate on getting the basics right, fine-tune the skills you already possess and show you some fresh ways of structuring your consultations to maximum effectiveness, both in the SCA and, afterwards, in real-life practice.

---

[7] In 2014, the British Association of Physicians of Indian Origin (BAPIO) took the RCGP and the General Medical Council to judicial review in the High Court, claiming that the difference in CSA pass rates between UK and non-UK medical graduates was a breach of equality legislation, and directly and indirectly indicated discrimination against international medical graduates and black and minority ethnic candidates. In his judgement, Mr. Justice Tilling dismissed the claims, ruling that 'The clinical skills assessment is a proportionate means of achieving the legitimate aim (of protecting the public),' and that 'There is no basis for contending that the small number who fail ultimately do so for any reason apart from their own shortcomings as prospective general practitioners.' But he also laid a duty on the RCGP to take whatever steps lay within its power to attempt to minimise the disadvantage at which overseas graduates found themselves.

> **EXAM POINT: If English is not your first language**
>
> It is inevitable, in an exam conducted in English and assessing fitness to practise in the UK, that candidates whose first language is not English face an additional challenge. In the SCA, everything possible is done to minimise any disadvantage to such candidates. Advice has been taken from experts in linguistics; every case scenario has been approved by an expert in equality, diversity and inclusion; and the role-players and examiners have all received ED&I training. Role-players will not have strong regional accents and will not use unnecessarily complex language or unfamiliar words. However, the time allowance of 12 minutes per case will not be extended to compensate for any language difficulties, unless they result from a condition for which a 'reasonable adjustment' is allowable. The RCGP website provides more details.

'Doctor-centred' or 'patient-centred'?

It is common to hear a distinction being made between 'doctor-centred' and 'patient-centred' styles of consulting, often with the implication that doctor-centred is bad (at least in general practice) and patient-centred is good. But there is some confusion about what these terms mean, and to think that one is good and the other bad is an over-simplification that can have damaging results.

'Doctor-centred' is the traditional way of practising medicine. We see it in its purest form in the 'medical model' most of us will have been taught at medical school. Starting with the patient's report of symptoms, the doctor leads the consultation through the time-honoured sequence:

History → *Examination* → *Investigations* → *Diagnosis* → *Treatment*

The doctor assumes the role of expert, not only in the diagnosis and management of disease but also in how this clinical expertise is to be applied to the particular circumstances of the individual patient. I use the word *assume* in both its meanings; the doctor assumes – takes on – the role of the expert, the repository of all relevant knowledge, and also assumes – takes it for granted – that the patient is happy to accept the role of passive beneficiary of the doctor's wisdom and will comply unquestioningly with whatever advice or treatment is handed down. The doctor decides what information is pertinent and obtains it using predominantly closed questions. The patient, by and large, should speak only when spoken to and should gratefully obey the doctor's instructions.

The doctor-centred method has its merits. It works well for purely physical diseases. It will usually succeed in serious, complicated or unusual cases, and is essential in life-threatening emergency situations. The patient of a doctor-centred clinician can be assured (if the doctor is competent and up-to-date) of the best possible evidence-based outcome.

But, as you know, an exclusively doctor-centred approach is not sustainable in general practice, where psychological, emotional, social, cultural and economic factors compound the problems patients bring to their GP, and even purely physical illness is modified in its presentation and impact by the different circumstances of each individual patient.

The term 'patient-centred' was first used in this context by Enid Balint in 1969[8] and has gradually become generally preferred as a style of consulting better suited to contemporary general practice in the UK. Patient-centredness incorporates two elements. The first is the importance of understanding illness as experienced from the patient's point of view – something about which they have thoughts and feelings, worries and expectations. The second is that the patient is an active participant in how the consultation is conducted, and especially in how management choices and decisions are made.

On the face of it, patient-centred consulting seems 'right' – an expression of the self-evident truth that both doctor and patient are human beings with similar rights and responsibilities – notwithstanding the knowledge gap that exists between them as far as medical matters are concerned. The shift from doctor-centred to patient-centred medicine can be seen as part of a general evolution in cultural norms towards a more egalitarian society, where everyone can access the world's information banks, and establishment figures, including professionals, can no longer command respect and influence as of right.

However, for all its OK-sounding vocabulary of 'partnership,' 'sharing' and 'involvement,' patient-centred consulting isn't right for everybody, or in all circumstances. A doctor whom most patients find refreshingly approachable, some will find evasive and unconfident. Another whose style can come across as paternalistic may, by some patients, be perceived as reassuring and trustworthy. Some patients, notably the elderly or those from some non-European backgrounds, are so used to 'the doctor as authority figure' that they are seriously unsettled by a doctor who appears over-friendly or who seems unwilling to tell them plainly what needs to be done. We should remember, too, that when people are ill or afraid, they tend to regress towards a more child-like state where they depend on the support of parental

---

[8] Balint E (1969) The possibility of patient-centred medicine. J R Coll Gen Pract. 17: 269–276. Enid was the wife of Hungarian psychoanalyst Michael Balint. Based at London's Tavistock Institute, together in the 1950s and 1960s they developed 'Balint groups' for GPs, which pioneered exploration of the doctor–patient relationship in general practice.

surrogates such as doctors, and that, at least in the short term, it can be appropriate for the doctor to take responsibility for decisions about their care.

The unsurprising conclusion is that a good GP can be doctor-centred or patient-centred as the patient or the circumstances require. If I board a plane to fly to Tokyo, I want control of the aircraft to be pilot-centred, not passenger-centred. But I want its destination to be passenger-centred, not pilot-centred. The ideal flight would be passenger-selected but pilot-flown. Be like that pilot. Get your patient safely to where they need to be, using all the knowledge, skills and experience at your command. That's what being patient-centred means.

The idea of patient-centredness can sometimes be misunderstood, especially by doctors whose background is in a healthcare system where it is an unfamiliar concept. The mistake is to think patient-centredness means that the patient is always right; that the patient must always get what they want; that they must always have choice and their choices must always be respected; and that their wishes or expectations must never be challenged. Equally mistaken is the idea that the doctor should never interrupt or cut the patient off in mid-narrative, or take active steps to control the format or duration of the consultation. Patient-centredness is not passivity. It is not enough for you to sit in your chair brimming with medical knowledge and full of benevolence towards your patient, and then just to hope that by some miracle the patient will give you exactly the information you need, in the right order, and within the time available, and will spontaneously depart at the end of their allotted time. They won't; and unless you do something about it, the consultation can easily drift or go around in circles, ultimately resulting in frustration and disappointment for both of you.

Patient-centredness means bringing all your skills – *all* your skills – to bear on the patient's problem, and that includes the consulting skills that enable you to bring the consultation to an effective conclusion in a limited time. In other words, it is acceptable – indeed, necessary – for you, on occasion, to take charge of the consultation's content and process and actively manage its timings, as long as you are doing so in what are genuinely the patient's best interests.

I suspect that most doctors, myself included, are probably closet doctor-centred consulters at heart. The doctor-centred medical model is, after all, the default approach most of us were trained in at medical school. If you're familiar with the basic ideas of Eric Berne's Transactional Analysis,[9] you

---

[9] Dating from the 1950s, Transactional Analysis is a psychoanalytic model of individuals and relationships. At any given moment, our thoughts, feelings and behaviour are in one of three 'ego states' – caring or critical Parent, emotional or immature Child, or logical rational Adult. The best-known popular introductory text, still well worth reading, is Eric Berne's Games People Play (New York: Ballantine Books, 1964).

will recognise the doctor–patient relationship in a doctor-centred consultation is that of parent to child, whereas a patient-centred consultation is more adult to adult. It takes a combination of determination, training, self-criticism and practice before we start to feel comfortable swopping the relative security of acting as the patient's parent or guardian in favour of behaving more like their colleague or collaborator. Sometimes, if we are inexperienced, and particularly when we are stressed, traces of persistent doctor-centredness show through our attempts to be patient-centred. We tend to interrupt the patient's narrative before it has had time to get going, often with closed 'medical' questions that cause the patient to tell a slightly different story from the one intended. We say things like, 'I think we should do X and Y – is that OK?' hoping that *Is that OK?* will suffice for 'sharing decision-making with the patient.' We pay lip service to 'checking the patient's understanding' by tacking on a perfunctory 'Any questions?' as we bring the consultation to a close.

No one ever said that consulting in general practice was going to be easy. But to think of it as a tension between doctor-centredness and patient-centredness doesn't help. I think what *does* help is an approach that combines the best of both – an approach that respects the patient's autonomy and uniqueness, while fully acknowledging the doctor's professional expertise. I think the ideal consultation is patient-focused and doctor-guided. And I think the three-part model I'm about to describe in detail is just that: **patient–focused, doctor–guided** (Figure 2.7).

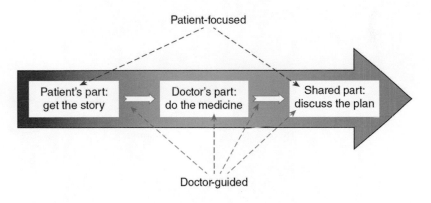

FIGURE 2.7

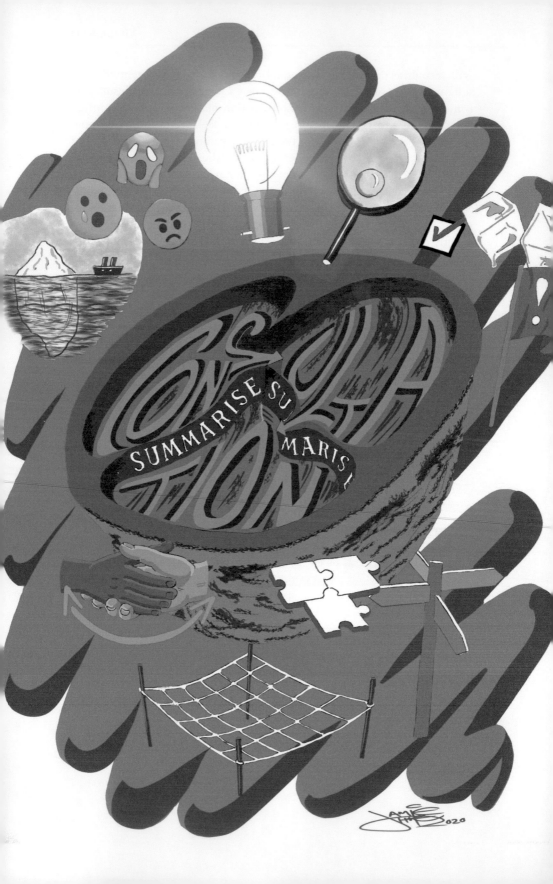

3

The consultation in a nutshell

As we begin to go into the detail of how to conduct a successful general practice consultation, take a moment to remember the essential simplicity of what you are trying to achieve. The patient comes to you with a problem and expects to leave with a plan for dealing with it. So your tasks are, first, to find out what the problem is – the *real* problem, the one you really need to concentrate on – and then to agree on a course of action that satisfies both of you (Figure 3.1).

The 'right' problem

A complication in this simple *What's-the-problem-and-what-are-we-going-to-do-about-it?* approach is that there are two, and sometimes three, versions of the problem. The first is the problem, as it appears from the patient's point of view at the start of the consultation. This is the version the patient will try to communicate to you in their opening narrative. The second is the problem as seen from your professional perspective and couched in medical terms. Very often, you will need to reframe or translate the patient's version into something you can 'do medicine' on. For example, the patient's opening complaint might be 'My guts aren't what they were, I just need a laxative'; but for you to take effective action, you need to interpret this as *Recent change of bowel habit.* Translating the problem into 'doctor-speak' is necessary in order for your medical training to kick in, alerting you to the possible significance of these symptoms and prompting you to the clinically appropriate response.

But quite often, a third version of the problem emerges after some discussion and exploration of the initial presentation, replacing it in the patient's mind as the accepted priority agenda. In the example I've given, you will

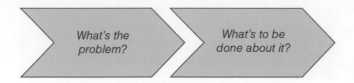

FIGURE 3.1

need to help the patient change the problem as they see it, from *I need a laxative* to *I have some possibly serious symptoms.* Unless you can do this, it will be difficult for you and the patient to agree on a management plan. Other examples of situations calling for what we might call 'secondary translation' of the presenting problem into the 'real' or underlying problem are:

- *hidden agenda*, e.g., the patient whose pain from a mild whiplash injury seems disproportionate until you discover that an insurance claim is pending;
- *the 'ticket of admission,'* e.g., a teenage girl who presents with mild acne but who 'really' wants contraception;
- *stress-related symptoms*, e.g., tension headaches in an overworked teacher;
- *psychosomatic or medically unexplained symptoms*, e.g., dyspareunia in a young woman who is the victim of domestic abuse.

In these examples, accepting and concentrating on the presenting version of the problem is likely to prove frustrating or disappointing to both doctor and patient. Although it can be tempting, in the interests of saving time, to take the patient's initial account of their problem at face value, this can be a false economy. Spending five minutes addressing the *wrong* problem will not save you from sooner or later having to deal with the *right* one. The message is that time spent in the early stages of the consultation on making sure you really *do* understand what the patient needs is a sound investment – provided, that is, that you don't spend so long doing so that you leave insufficient time for the *What-are-we-going-to-do-about-it?* management part of the consultation.

A typical consultation

Figure 3.2 illustrates what happens in a typical general practice consultation. In the British NHS, this will last, on average, about 10 minutes, plus or minus a bit. In the SCA exam, it will be exactly 720 seconds!

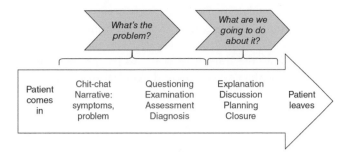

FIGURE 3.2

The arrow represents the period of time from when the patient comes in and the consultation starts until they leave, about 10 minutes later. It will usually begin with a brief exchange of social chit-chat: a greeting and a confirmatory exchange of names if the doctor and patient haven't met before. Very common is this:

Doctor: 'I'm sorry you've been waiting.'
Patient: 'I'm sorry to trouble you.'

Patients generally understand that they are expected to start by telling the doctor why they have come. Sometimes they might need a prompt such as, 'How can I help?' or 'What can I do for you today?' What the patient then offers is usually a story, a narrative. The story will include some of their symptoms or details of whatever is worrying them, but these tend to be embedded within a discursive account of the circumstances when the patient realised there was a problem. Patients don't always present a concise, medically focused statement such as, 'My right knee has been increasingly painful for six weeks.'[1] It is more likely that what you will be told is, 'Anyway, last week, I was standing at the bus stop, waiting for a bus to go down to see Mother – she's in the hospital with her heart, did you know? – and my knees were really giving me gyp. I mean, you have to expect it at my age, I suppose, but if it's going to be like this once she comes home, and I'll be up and down stairs … So I thought, best get something sorted out.'

---

[1] In SCA cases, the simulated patient often does begin with a concise opening statement, as the role-players are trained to start the consultation in the same way with every candidate in the interests of consistency and fairness. It's then up to you to get them to expand on it, probably with some open questions.

As you listen to the patient's narrative, you start to get ideas about what the main problem might be. Some of your thoughts will be medical: *Is this arthritis? Probably osteo, but remember the other causes of knee pain.* Reading between the lines, you will also have picked up some possible pointers to the patient's concerns and expectations: *Is she worried about her ability to look after an elderly relative? Does she want symptom relief, or a referral, or a package of support for her mother? Is she worried that she too might develop heart problems?* These are important questions, but the patient may well not have supplied the answers to them in her story. In order to come up with an appropriate management plan, you need to know more than you have so far been told. So, once you have listened to the patient's initial narrative, you ask questions to obtain the additional information you need. *Are any joints other than the knee involved? Have you tried any over-the-counter medicines? When will your mother be discharged from hospital? Will you be her principal carer? How is your mood? Are you worried about the future?* And if it is clinically relevant, you might want to supplement your verbal questions with a physical examination; in this case, of the knees and other joints, looking for signs of local or generalised osteoarthritis or other causes of arthropathy.

So far, the consultation has been concerned with data-gathering. You are building a picture of the patient's problem by putting together information of two distinct types. The first is the information the patient explicitly tells you in their opening story, either unprompted or with a little encouragement from you. We could call this 'patient-volunteered' information. The second is the additional information that the patient provides only if you take the initiative and ask for it. This second type, which would include the findings of any physical examination, we could call 'doctor-prompted' information.

Now that your data-gathering is complete, you are in a position to answer the question *What's the problem?* You can make a 'good enough to work with' assessment of the patient's main reason for consulting you. Your overall assessment might include a physical diagnosis or a differential diagnosis. But, because you are a GP caring for the whole patient, it should also incorporate psychological, emotional and social dimensions. For instance, you might decide that the patient I have just described does indeed have a moderate degree of osteoarthritis, but that her chief worry is that her bad knee could affect her ability to care for her ageing mother. In purely physical terms, the provisional diagnosis is osteoarthritis, but your assessment as a GP extends beyond this to take in its impact on her role in the family and on her own state of mind.

At this point, the consultation changes gear and moves on to the *What-are-we-going-to-do-about-it?* stage of decision-making and management planning. Your goal now becomes to agree on the best action plan – one that, so far as possible, has the best chance of satisfying the patient's needs and expectations and also of meeting your own standards of good practice. In most cases (emergency situations being an exception), you will now be explaining your assessment of the problem; presenting and discussing the realistic treatment options; and allowing the patient to contribute to discussion, state their own preferences, and exercise choice insofar as is possible. In the case of the woman with the painful knees, you might be suggesting some X-rays, discussing the relative merits of analgesics or nonsteroidal anti-inflammatory medication, and outlining what forms of help might be available as her mother becomes increasingly dependent. Once a mutually acceptable plan has been agreed upon, you will probably need to spell out in detail how it is to be implemented, including any plans for follow-up or dealing with any unexpected developments ('safety-netting'). You will check to make sure the patient understands the plan and give her the chance to ask any questions.

All that now remains is to close the consultation in a friendly way, such as, 'Come and see me again when the X-ray results are back. And we can discuss what support can be arranged for when your Mum comes out of hospital.'

The three-part consultation

Remember: the overarching aim of the consultation is to convert a problem into a plan; and, at its simplest, the process for doing so has two stages.

First, identify the problem that needs your attention.

Then, work out what is to be done about it.

But this is a bit *too* simple. As the physicist Albert Einstein supposedly said, 'Everything should be made as simple as possible – but no simpler.' Let me explain the difficulty and then tell you how it can be overcome.

As we discussed a couple of sections ago, the two people involved – the patient and you – have different perspectives on how they see the problem and what they think is relevant information about it. The patient's version, the version they first describe when invited to tell you about it, is inevitably highly subjective. Some of the points they bring out will be things that matter to them; others will be what they *imagine* will matter to *you*. Consciously or unconsciously, they will emphasise some aspects of their story and suppress others. You will be offered a mixture of facts, thoughts and feelings, all of which are expressed in lay (or sometimes pseudo-medical) language.

You, on the other hand, need objective data and reliable information in order to understand the situation in terms that you, as a medical professional, can analyse, interpret and act upon. Being a good GP, you of course also want to understand the 'softer' aspects of the patient's problem – the context, implications and effects that the patient knows about, but you, at least to start with, don't. The trouble is, early in the consultation, you can't always tell what is reliable and relevant information and what is irrelevant padding. You can't always tell whether an apparently inconsequential remark is indeed of no consequence or whether, in fact, it is a significant cue to some unexpressed but important agenda. And if you interrupt the patient, who might be in full flow, whenever a question occurs to you, you can easily put them off their stride and cause the consultation to stall.

So what's the better way?

The 'simple but not *too* simple' answer is this:

At the start of the consultation, split the task of data-gathering into two parts. The first part – the Patient's part – is when you concentrate on getting the patient's version of the problem as fully as you can. The second part – the Doctor's part – is when you obtain whatever additional information you need in order to complete your professional assessment of the situation (Figure 3.3).

In other words, think of 'getting the patient's take on the situation' and 'formulating your own medical understanding of it' as two separate stages in your data-gathering. And let the patient go first.

Why make this clear distinction between information that the patient volunteers and information that you actively seek? And why does the patient get to go first? It sounds like a recipe, if the patient is vague or garrulous, for the consultation to drag on forever.

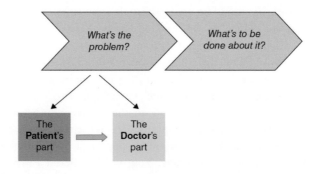

FIGURE 3.3

Yes, it could, unless – unless you have the necessary time-management skills to prevent it and make sure that you can wind up the Patient's part and move on to the Doctor's part in a timely and effective fashion. Making the transition from Patient's part to Doctor's part is what that green arrow represents in Figure 3.3. Don't worry, I'll show you some ways of doing it later on in this book. Remember, this is going to be a patient-focused *but doctor-guided* way of consulting.

In practically every consultation, after any brief chit-chat and possibly a 'How can I help you?' from the doctor, the patient begins by making an opening statement. Quite often, this will have been thought about in advance and silently rehearsed in the waiting room.[2] It represents the patient's chosen way of raising the concerns that have prompted the consultation. But it is only the first few lines in what they expect to be a longer narrative, which will (if you give them the chance) reveal a more comprehensive version of their agenda. It is in your interests to get the patient as quickly and efficiently as you can into *telling-the-doctor-all-about-it* mode. And the best way to do this is for you to pay wholehearted, non-intrusive attention. The patient needs not only to be listened to, but also to *know* that they are being listened to. It's largely a question of mindset. To keep the patient in 'telling' mode, your own mindset needs to be one of curiosity: attentive to and genuinely interested in what you are being told; open-minded and uncritical; alert to any pointers in the patient's language or behaviour to additional dimensions to their problem.

As you listen to the patient's opening narrative, encouraging and clarifying it as necessary, inevitably you find yourself thinking 'medically' about what you are hearing. Possible diagnoses, possible explanations and possible next courses of action: all start to occur to you. You realise you are going to need more information than the patient has so far given you. You may want to know specific details of symptoms, their timing and effects. There may be 'red flag' questions you will need to ask. You may have a sense of needing to explore more deeply the patient's worries or expectations. And, depending on the nature of the case, you might anticipate that a physical examination of some kind is going to be called for.

But as far as possible, during the Patient's part, you will keep these thoughts to yourself. You put your questions and your medical agenda on hold for the time being, so as not to disrupt the patient's 'protected time' at the beginning of the consultation. The time to ask all these

---

[2] In my book *The Inner Consultation*, I call this the 'opening gambit,' analogous to the first moves in a game of chess.

supplementary questions and to acquire all this additional information comes next, in the Doctor's part. The Doctor's part is *your* protected space in the consultation – the time when *you* take the lead, when *you* steer the conversation to find out what *you* want to know. The Doctor's part is your 'filling in the gaps' time.

When you transition to the Doctor's part, the mindsets need to change. You need to switch from 'listening' mode to 'questioning' mode, and the patient correspondingly has to move out of 'free-narrative' mode and into 'answering-questions' mode.

You might think it's possible, even desirable, to let these shifts in mindset – the doctor switching between listener and interrogator, the patient between storyteller and question-answerer – alternate freely as the patient's problem is gradually revealed and explored. But it's really hard to get the timing right. For two people to coordinate rapid shifts in who is leading the conversation, it requires a sophisticated degree of rapport between them. You see it between lovers or close friends, but doctor and patient are seldom so attuned to the subtleties of each other's communication cues. In consultations that go badly, you often find doctor and patient getting into a battle for control of the information flow, with the patient trying to tell their story in their own way and the doctor trying to take over and convert it into the 'medical' version they would rather be hearing. The result is confusion, misunderstanding and frustration. In the data-gathering stage of the consultation, it is much neater and more effective to make a clear demarcation between patient-led disclosure and doctor-led enquiry. Cross–contamination between the Patient's part and Doctor's part usually ends in a muddle.

By the end of the Doctor's part, which can include a physical examination if this is indicated, you should have enough data to formulate a version of the patient's problem that you as a medical professional can work with. How you convert information into a diagnosis or an insight into the patient's problem is something I *can't* help you with. If your knowledge of clinical medicine isn't adequate, or if your understanding of human nature doesn't go deep enough, no amount of consulting skills will be an acceptable substitute.

Assuming, however, that you *do* now have a working appreciation of what the problem is that needs your attention, it's time to draw a line under your information-gathering. It is often a good idea at this stage to summarise the story so far; in other words, to offer the patient a short recap of the key points you have picked up from their story, together with your own interpretation and assessment of what the problem is. A good summary is reassuring to the patient, confirming that what they wanted to tell you has

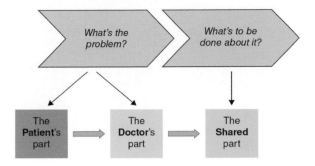

FIGURE 3.4

been heard and understood, and also to yourself, so that you can be confident that you haven't missed anything important.

Now it's time to move on to the final *What-are-we-going-to-do-about-it?* phase of the consultation, which I'm calling the Shared part (Figure 3.4). This is the decision-making and action-planning part of the consultation, where doctor and patient collaborate and agree on a management plan they are both happy with – the patient because they recognise it meets their needs and the doctor because it constitutes a good piece of medicine. It's also the hardest part to do well, and the part where most marks are lost in the SCA. It's where the difference between a doctor-centred doctor and a patient-centred one is most clearly seen. And it's the part that suffers most under time pressure, both in the exam and in real-life practice.

I hope you can now see how and why the simple two-stage consultation process has expanded to three parts. If this idea is new to you, please take a few moments as you read this to stop and think about it. I'm suggesting that you keep a clear distinction in your mind between the problem as the patient sees it and the problem as *you* need to see it in medical terms. I'm suggesting that you investigate these two perspectives separately, concentrating first on the patient's version and saving most of your medical questions until the patient has had their say. When you think you're clear about what the problem is, confirm it with the patient and then move on to consider what is to be done about it. Before the consultation finishes, make sure the patient is as happy with the management plan as *you* are. And I'm suggesting that the responsibility for making sure the consultation moves seamlessly from the Patient's to the Doctor's to the Shared part is yours and yours alone. In Figure 3.4, you're in charge of the green arrows.

Here (Figure 3.5) is a visual summary of where we've got to so far.

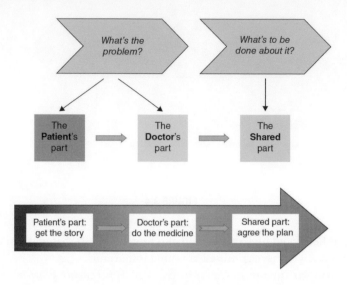

FIGURE 3.5

More about the Patient's part

A few years ago, I learned a humbling lesson from an unexpected teacher. I had developed a pain in my left ankle, just above the medial malleolus, which I was genuinely at a loss to account for. It got steadily worse, so when it started to keep me awake at night, I decided there was nothing for it but to consult an orthopaedic surgeon – someone previously unknown to me. I'm ashamed to say that such were my preconceptions about orthopaedic surgeons that I had no high expectations of his consultation skills. Never mind, I thought, I just want to know what's the matter with my ankle. When I entered his room, it was clear he didn't realise I was a doctor; he'd not even read the GP's letter. But his first words to me were these: 'Tell me what you want me to hear, in your own words.' *Tell me what you want me to hear, in your own words.* I have never before or since heard a better way of beginning a consultation. What he seemed to be saying was, 'I know you've got something on your mind you want to tell me about. OK, I'm listening; go for it' (Figure 3.6).[3]

---

[3] The diagnosis turned out to be tibialis posterior tenosynovitis, brought on by long-distance running with flat feet. More importantly, I also learned that GPs don't have a monopoly where patient-centredness and skilful communication are concerned.

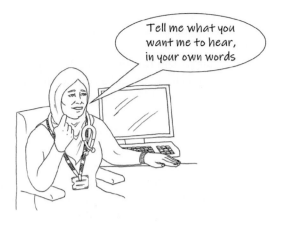

FIGURE 3.6

Whether or not you use the surgeon's words *verbatim* in your own consultations, the attitude that came across from him is exactly the right one to have at the beginning of the Patient's part. Every patient who consults you brings a potential story with them. Or, in fact, they bring *several* potential stories with them; your role in the Patient's part is to help the various stories get told.

The first story is the one the patient has planned on telling you – the one that quite often they will have been rehearsing on the way to see you. It might be concise and to the point, e.g., 'I've been getting indigestion for the last three months,' or 'I'm worried about my husband's drinking.' Your response to stories that begin like this will usually be along the lines of 'Tell me more …' Other stories begin more hesitantly and become vague or rambling, e.g., 'I'm probably just wasting your time, and you must get sick of seeing people like me, but, well, I'm just not right.' In these situations, your role is to help the patient find a focus for their story without over-influencing it or getting too medical too soon.

No matter how it starts, the patient's story will include something about the symptoms or concerns that have made them come to see you. These early pointers to the consultation's agenda will usually be embedded within a narrative describing other aspects of the patient's life and experience. You might be told, for instance, how they first came to think there was a problem; or how they have been affected by it; or what they think might be causing it; or what they think it might lead to. It's impossible for us human beings to encounter a problem without our imagination coming up with thoughts about why it has happened, worries about potential consequences, and fantasies about possible solutions. All these possibilities will be lurking within the patient's opening narrative; and the well-known trio of Ideas, Concerns and Expectations reminds us of the importance of discovering them.[4]

Behind the story the patient first tells you, there might be another one – a 'story in waiting' as it were. It might be a more comprehensive version of the first, or even a different problem altogether, which the patient *could* tell you with a bit of prompting and if they get the chance. A common example is the 'And another thing' patient, who has a list of problems but doesn't say so at the outset. Another would be the 'ticket of admission' scenario, such as the girl presenting with mild acne who waits to see how you deal with this before asking about contraception, which is the 'real' reason she has come.

There may even be another story buried even deeper – the one the patient fully intended *not* to tell you; something about which they perhaps feel ashamed, or embarrassed, or foolish, or guilty. The woman who tells you she is worried about her husband's drinking, for example, might be a secret victim of domestic violence and having an extra-marital affair, neither of which facts did she intend to mention. But if you create the right atmosphere of trust and give her the right encouragement, she might feel safe enough to divulge them, thereby giving you a more complete picture of the situation you are being asked to help with.

Everything you say and do in the Patient's part should be aimed primarily at helping the patient tell their story – the 'surface' story at least, and as much as is feasible of any 'deeper' ones. The key thoughts for you to keep in mind are *What is the story this person needs to tell me? And how can I help them tell it?* Resist the temptation to interrupt or to steer the narrative in any particular direction. This is the patient's protected time to use as they see fit. For the time being, keep quiet about any medical thoughts that start to occur to you. You will have plenty of opportunity to voice them in the next part of the consultation, the Doctor's part. By the end of the Patient's part (Figure 3.7), you should aim to have a fair idea of:

- how the patient sees the problem,
- what they want from the consultation, and
- why they want it.

And how will you know whether your ideas are right? In a word – summarise. Give a succinct summary of what you have understood so far, and let the patient correct or amplify it if necessary.

---

[4] I'll have more to say about 'ICE' later. For now, remember it's not just a piece of consultation-speak jargon; it's a reminder to try to understand the problem from the patient's point of view.

The PATIENT'S part
'What is the story this patient needs to tell?'

• The story they planned to tell you
• Symptoms, problems, worries
• How they are affected by the problem
• Ideas, concerns & expectations
• The story they *could* tell you with a bit of prompting
• What do you think the patient wants?
• And why do they want it?

FIGURE 3.7

More about the Doctor's part

In the Patient's part, it was the patient who was in charge of the flow of information. The patient chose which story to tell and how to tell it. Your role was to assist and encourage the telling, without trying to impose your own ideas of what you wanted to hear. As you listened, you will have started to think of various hypotheses as to what, medically speaking, might be going on. And there will be a number of questions you want to ask: to clarify facts, gather evidence about possible diagnoses, or test your interpretation of events. *'She could be anaemic, or hypothyroid. I need to ask if there's a family history of thyroid disease. But she sounds quite depressed. I'm not surprised, with a marriage like that …'* But, so as not to disrupt the patient's narrative, you have refrained from interrupting and put your doctor-led agenda on hold.

Now, however, in the Doctor's part, it becomes *your* turn to take the lead in data-gathering, and pursue whatever additional information *you* need to help you come to a medical assessment of the problem. It is now *you* in the driving seat. This is *your* protected time in the consultation. The questions you ask now are the ones *you* want to know the answer to. You switch from being an interested listener to an active investigator; and the patient correspondingly switches from being a storyteller to a witness, answering your questions.

So the Doctor's part is when you get to:

• enquire about specific details of the problem or symptoms that were not clear from the patient's account, such as timings, type of pain, self-medication, etc.;

• ask any other medically relevant questions, such as symptoms in other body systems, past medical history, medication history, family and social circumstances;

The DOCTOR'S part
'What more do I need to know?'

- Clarification of the symptoms/problem
- Other medically-relevant questions
- 'Red flag' questions
- Exploration of cues or hidden agenda
- Ideas, concerns & expectations
- Physical examination, if indicated
- Diagnosis, differential diagnosis or 'working assessment'
- Summarise

FIGURE 3.8

- ask about 'red flag' symptoms, if they are clinically indicated to exclude serious disease;
- clarify the patient's ideas, concerns and expectations, if they have not emerged during the Patient's part;
- explore any cues you might have picked up from the patient's narrative suggesting there could be undisclosed issues or hidden agenda;
- carry out a physical examination if it is clinically indicated;
- confirm that you have correctly identified the key features of the patient's problem, perhaps by summarising the story and the facts as you understand them.

The key thought to keep in mind during the Doctor's part is: *'What more information do I need in order to make a proper professional assessment of the problem?'* Hopefully, by the end of the Doctor's part you should be in a position to make a provisional diagnosis or a differential diagnosis, or (failing that) will have a clear enough understanding of the problem to allow you to come up with a possible plan of action (Figure 3.8).

And how do you let the patient know that you think you understand the problem and are ready to move on and discuss management? In a word – summarise.

More about the Shared part

Ideally, the consultation should end with two happy people. The patient should leave feeling satisfied, knowing that they have been helped, and the doctor should be left feeling quietly pleased with a job well done. So the key thought to guide you during this final phase of the consultation is *'What plan of action will best satisfy the expectations of both of us – me and the patient?'*

Usually, at the end of the Doctor's part, when you have gathered as much information as realistically possible and have had a chance to get your medical thoughts in order, you will have in mind what we might call 'Plan A.' Plan A would be the management plan you would make if it were left entirely to you – your personal recommendation as to the best way forward.

In past times (and still in some healthcare systems), when a heavily doctor-centred style of medicine was the norm, your Plan A would have been non-negotiable. You would have made your management decisions, and the patient would have accepted them unquestioningly. That authoritarian approach is now history, and few lament its passing. Nowadays, we (and that includes the SCA examiners) expect decisions to be made collaboratively, with doctor and patient each making their contribution. After all, the doctor may be an expert in medicine, but the patient is an expert in his or her own life. In a more consumerist society, we all expect to have a say in decisions that affect us and to exercise a degree of choice where there is more than one option available.

So in the Shared part (Figure 3.9), doctor and patient are working their way towards a mutually acceptable outcome, which may or may not be the provisional Plan A you first thought of. Indeed, even if it *is* Plan A that is finally agreed upon, the patient needs to feel involved in its formulation if they are to feel satisfied and committed to it. However, it is easy to have this patient-centred approach as an aspiration, but not so easy to carry out in real life. Shared decision-making is likely to involve you in:

- explaining your assessment of the problem to the patient in language they can readily understand;
- discussing the factors that, in your opinion, might affect management;

The SHARED part
'What management plan will we both be happy with?'

- Explaining
- Discussing
- Respecting patient's preferences and health beliefs
- Considering options
- Collaborative decision-making
- Action planning
- Checking for understanding
- Safety-netting and follow-up plans

FIGURE 3.9

- putting together and explaining a comprehensive plan of action that accords as far as possible with current guidelines and standards of good practice;

- finding out if your patient has any preferences or health beliefs that might affect any management decisions and paying them appropriate respect during discussion;

- considering any alternative options to your preferred plan, including any suggestions by the patient;

- involving the patient in making decisions as much or as little as they wish and respecting their wishes and opinions;

- making sure that the patient understands and accepts the management plan and has an opportunity to ask any questions;

- making appropriate plans for follow-up, including 'safety-netting' to cater for any unexpected developments.

Transitions – keeping the consultation on track

To summarise: you begin the consultation by allowing and encouraging the patient to give as full an account as possible of the problem as they see it. You then take the lead, fleshing out the patient's story by eliciting whatever additional information you need to form your medical assessment. This done, data-gathering being complete and your working assessment of the problem being clear in your mind, you move on to jointly devising a management plan that is medically sound and also acceptable to the patient.

OK so far?

But there is one final element I need to introduce before we can get into the details of how to make this neat and convenient theory work out in real life.

There are two places in the consultation where things have to change and the consultation has to take a different turn. One part of the consultation has to come to an end and make way for the next. After the Patient's part has run its course, a line has to be drawn under the patient's narrative because it is time to move on to the Doctor's part. This transition from the Patient's to the Doctor's part is shown as Transition 1 in Figure 3.10. A little later, after you have finished the Doctor's part, there needs to be a second transition, Transition 2, when you move from data-gathering into the management planning of the Shared part.

These transitions from one part to the next at the appropriate time are important for keeping the consultation on track and completing it in the

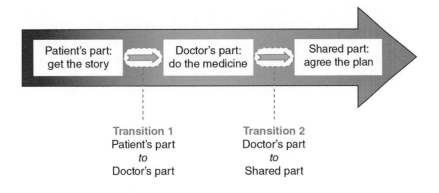

FIGURE 3.10

time available. If Transition 1 doesn't happen, you could get bogged down, particularly with a talkative patient, in a rambling or repetitious recital producing little worthwhile information, and never get around to your own doctor-led questioning. Likewise, towards the end of the Doctor's part, you have to stop gathering information, settle for what you've got, 'change gear,' and, at Transition 2, move the consultation on into its action-planning stage.

You can't assume that these transitions will happen by themselves. If necessary, you have to *make* them happen. It's not enough for you to sit in your chair, brim-full of knowledge and patient-centred goodwill, and just hope the patient's narrative will be self-limiting and that the patient will, after three minutes or so, say to you, 'Well that's enough from me, doctor; I expect you've got some questions of your own to ask me now.' When it's time to move on to the Doctor's part, you have to be able in effect to say to the patient (though of course you won't use these exact words!), 'Stop now, it's *my* turn.'

Later, at Transition 2, you have to be able in effect to say to the patient (and why *not* use these exact words, or something very like them?), 'Well, I think we've got all the information we need to understand what the problem is; so let's now move on and talk about what's to be done about it.'

Transitions are when, if necessary, you take control of the consultation process and 'steer' it in order to keep it moving smoothly through the *Patient's part → Doctor's part → Shared part* sequence. If you misunderstand what patient-centredness means and think it's unprofessional to ever assert your own will over the patient's, you may have some difficulty accepting the importance of transitions. On the contrary, it's unprofessional *not* to.

You have limited time in which to do your best to bring each consultation to a successful conclusion.[5] To do this, it's your duty to use all the skills at your disposal, including what you know about how to structure and run an effective and efficient consultation. Transitions are an essential part of this. Later in this book, I'll explain some ways of steering the consultation that, although 'doctor-guided,' are nonetheless genuinely patient-focused.

Summary – the consultation in a nutshell

I've tried to capture the essence of this chapter in Figure 3.11. Don't just glance at it and say, 'Yes, got that.' Really look at it and make sure you understand what each element is describing. Try to get a sense of how your mindset moves and flows, from being curious about your patient's story to the analytical thought processes of the skilled clinician, and finally to a collaborative 'What will work for both of us?' And try to imagine being able to keep track of how the consultation is unfolding so that, if necessary, you can make mid-course corrections to keep it going in the right direction.

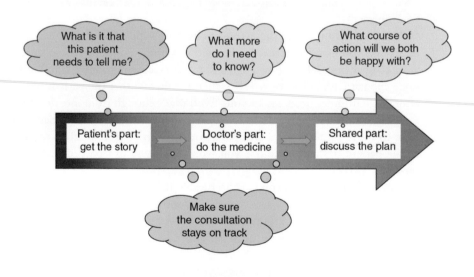

FIGURE 3.11

---

[5] In the SCA, of course, you have exactly 12 minutes per consultation. What you haven't done by the end of this time, you won't be given any credit for. So time management and process management are even more important under exam conditions.

This is 'the consultation in a nutshell,' and it's the framework around which the rest of this book is structured. Everything that follows will make more sense and be easier to remember if you can see how it fits into the overall picture.

The important features of this way of thinking about the consultation are as follows:

- Take time to identify the 'right' problem before moving on to management.
- Start by getting the patient's account of the problem as fully as you can before weighing in with your own questions.
- Try to keep the patient in 'telling-the-doctor-all-about-it' mode as long as possible at the start of the consultation.
- Aim to keep a clear separation between the three parts of the consultation. Avoid jumping backwards and forwards between them. Try not to contaminate the Patient's part with questions that really belong in the Doctor's part.
- The time you spend in each part will vary from case to case. But the sequence *Patient's part → Doctor's part → Shared part* should *not* vary.
- Judge the right moment to make the transition from one part to the next. Don't be afraid to steer the consultation if you feel it's necessary.

Before we move on

Although I hope that what I've written so far makes sense, what really matters is how it works out in practice. This will be the emphasis of the next chapter of this book, *Making a success of the three-part consultation*.

But before we plunge into the details, remind yourself of why you're bothering to try and get into good consulting habits. What we're talking about is a general strategy for being helpful to someone who needs your expertise – a patient who comes to you with a problem and hopes to leave with a plan. The single most important part of problem-solving is to make sure you properly identify the most important features of the problem. The best way to start is to try and understand the situation from the patient's point of view. And the best way of getting inside the patient's skin, as it were, is to pay them your very best attention while they're telling you about their problem. That means you should start the consultation in a state of alert curiosity: *What is it that this person has come to tell me?* If you listen attentively, and encourage, and don't interrupt, and don't change the subject, and don't prematurely jump to conclusions, you'll soon find out.

However, listening and understanding aren't enough. They *might* be if you were the patient's parent or best friend or counsellor. But you're not; you're their doctor. You're being consulted not just because you provide a listening ear but because you have medical expertise from which the patient hopes to benefit. And you know that in order for the patient to gain maximum benefit, you need reliable information: information that might not emerge from the patient's story and that you might therefore have to ask them for. So when you reach the Doctor's part of the consultation, your mindset shifts from 'curious listener' to 'analytic investigator.'

The combination of curiosity followed by analysis provides you with the best available information on which to base your assessment of *'What's the problem and what could be done about it?'* Converting *'What could be done about it?'* into *'What shall we actually agree to do about it?'* calls for a second change of mindset on your part – from 'analytic' to 'collaborative.'

Are you capable of being sometimes curious, sometimes analytic and sometimes collaborative? Of course you are, in your personal life outside medicine. When someone in your family has a bad day, you want to hear about it. When your car starts making funny noises, you try to figure out what it might be. When you're planning your summer holiday, you discuss it with the other people involved before deciding. All you have to do is bring into the consulting room the same qualities of caring, insight, respect and cooperation that you give to your family and friends without a second thought.

What's that? This *Patient's part → Doctor's part → Shared part* approach is what you're doing already? Your consultations already go through the sequence of taking a history, asking questions and sharing the decision-making? If that's true – wonderful! But *is* it true or as true as you think?

I have a challenge for you. If your consultations are truly in the *'three parts with transitions'* format, I ought to be able to interrupt you at any point and ask you which part of the consultation you are in – and you ought to know. You ought to be able to say, for example, 'We're still in the Patient's part; I haven't started the Doctor's part yet.' Or, 'I'm just wrapping up the Doctor's part and ready to move on to the Shared part.' So here's the challenge: watch a video recording of some of your consultations and see whether you can clearly distinguish between patient-led story-telling, doctor-led data-gathering and collaborative action-planning. If you're anything like the rest of us, there will be times when you cut across the patient's narrative to ask a question that might have been better saved until the Doctor's part. Or sometimes, during the Shared part, you may well find yourself flipping back and asking something that could have been clarified during the Patient's part.

I'm not challenging you on these points in order to be critical. And I certainly don't mean to imply that any departure from the 'three parts' approach is any kind of failure on your part. The 'three parts' approach, like any consultation model, is only a suggested framework, not a rule or a prescription. What I *am* trying to do is encourage you to cultivate self-awareness – the ability to monitor what's happening in the consultation *while* it's happening. Self-awareness gives you insight and manoeuvrability.

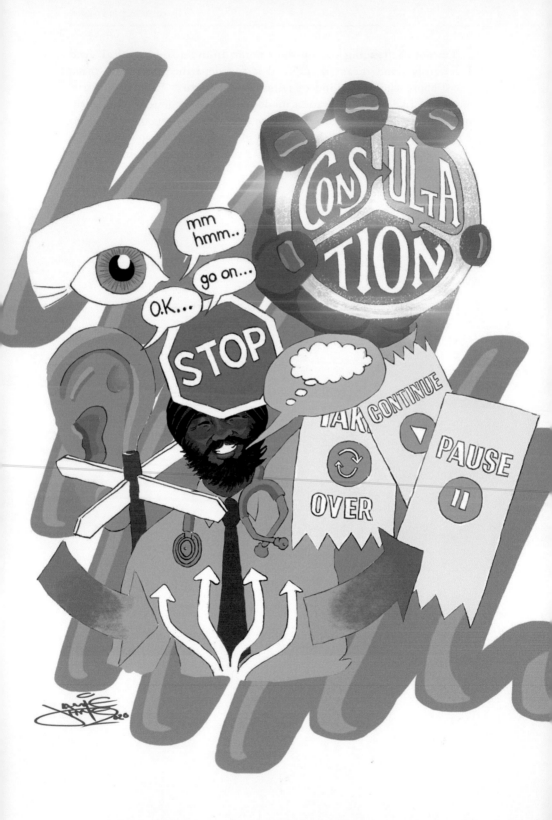

4

Making a success of the three-part consultation

My aim in this chapter is to show you in detail how to put the three-part approach into practice. We'll take the three parts of the consultation in turn and see how to make a success of each of them. And we'll look at how to transition cleanly and elegantly from one part to the next so that you develop a fluent and efficient consulting style that will leave the SCA examiners in no doubt that you know what you're doing, and which will stand you in good stead throughout your general practice career. Along the way, I'll remind you of some familiar consulting skills and also introduce you to a few others – such as using 'receipts' and 'thinking aloud' – which, once you've got them under your belt and they've become second nature to you, will boost your confidence that you can handle any challenge your consultations present (Figure 4.1).

Incidentally, I have called this chapter *Making a success …* in order to emphasise that the responsibility for bringing the consultation to a successful outcome rests with you – the doctor. A successful consultation doesn't just happen; you have to *make* it happen. Managing the consultation for maximum effectiveness is as much a professional competence as recognising papilloedema or taking a blood pressure.

> *The most important thing is to find out what is the most important thing.*
>
> **Shunryu Suzuki (1904–1971)**
> Japanese Zen Master

DOI: 10.1201/9781032619200-4

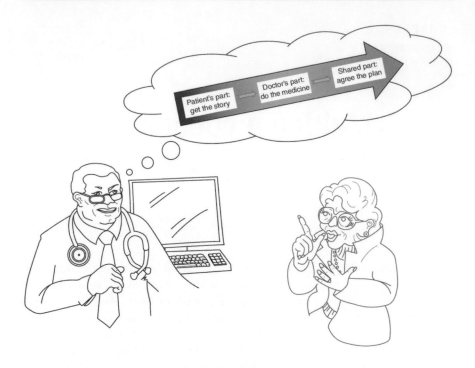

FIGURE 4.1

Making a success of the Patient's part

Everything you say and do at the start of the consultation should be directed towards understanding what, from the patient's point of view, is bothering them; what is bothering them the *most*; and what, if you could help with it, would give the greatest relief (Figure 4.2).

The more thoroughly you can understand the patient's 'take' on their problem, the easier you make the task of completing your data–gathering in the Doctor's part. It's very tempting, when you're anxious or short of time, to skimp on the Patient's part in your eagerness to get on to your doctor-led home territory. But try to resist this temptation. Time spent in the Patient's part saves you time later. It increases your chances of identifying the *right* problem. And it means that the questions you ask and the examination you perform in the Doctor's part will be more relevant and focused.

'Telling-the-doctor-all-about-it' mode

A huge amount of valuable information is potentially to be found in the story the patient first presents for your attention. As well as with the factual

The PATIENT'S part
'What is the story this patient needs to tell?'

- The story they planned to tell you
- Symptoms, problems, worries
- How they are affected by the problem
- Ideas, concerns & expectations
- The story they *could* tell you with a bit of prompting
- What do you think the patient wants?
- And why do they want it?

FIGURE 4.2

details of the problem, the patient's opening narrative – what they say and how they say it – can give you important pointers to their priority concerns, their feelings, their health beliefs and their expectations. It is in your interests, therefore, to get the patient as quickly as possible into 'telling-the-doctor-all-about-it' mode. And you need to have your attention turned up to maximum sensitivity so as not to miss the significant information being offered to you.

Some people are naturally extroverts and readily forthcoming. They feel comfortable talking about themselves, so when they consult as patients, they settle very easily into 'telling-you-all-about-it' mode. Indeed, you may find it necessary, in the Patient's part, to rein them in to some extent so that they don't lose track of their own story. Others are by nature more introverted, reticent and passive. As patients, they are more comfortable answering questions than volunteering information. For you, the challenge is to encourage and coax them out of 'answering' and into 'narrative' mode by, for example, using open invitations such as my orthopaedic surgeon's 'Tell me what you want me to hear, in your own words.'

The opening moments of the consultation are crucial to its success. Get the beginning right, and the rest of the consultation tends to go well. But if it gets off to a bad start, it can be very difficult to rescue it and get things back on track. It's important, therefore, for you to appear welcoming, attentive and interested from the outset, so that the patient feels encouraged to speak freely.

Greetings and introductions

Although from your point of view, the consultation only begins when the patient enters the room, the patient has been thinking about it for some time previously. They have been imagining how it will go, thinking what to say and wondering what *you* will say. It's as if, for the patient, the consultation has already begun. So everything you say or do, even the briefest of greetings, comes as something of an interruption to a story that, in their mind's ear, they are already telling. And no one likes to be interrupted in mid-story.

On the other hand, entering a doctor's consulting room and being expected to reveal what might be sensitive personal information is bound to be a bit intimidating. Your patient might need a little time to size you up and for their initial anxiety to subside before they can get on with their agenda for the consultation.

What you say by way of greeting and introduction needs, therefore, to be as non-intrusive as possible. At the same time, it should help put the patient at ease and signal that you're ready to hear what they have to tell you. In short, say as little as you can get away with – but say it encouragingly.

We all have little rituals for how we usually begin our consultations. A typical one might be, 'Hello, come in. Mrs X? I'm Doctor Y. How can I help you today?' Something like this is a sufficient signal that the patient can begin their opening narrative. But some trainee GPs – and I don't know whether it stems from unnecessary status anxiety or from misplaced advice from their trainers, aware that they are seeing many patients for the first time – are wont to overdo their introductory greeting and deliver a speech such as the following. (I exaggerate slightly to make the point.) 'Hello, I'm Doctor So-and-So, I'm a trainee in the practice, my trainer is Dr Z. I'm on the local training scheme. We've not met before, but I'm going to be here for the next twelve months, so we'll have a chance to get to know each other. Except on Wednesday afternoons, because that's the half-day release scheme. Anyway, it's nice to meet you, and' (*gasp*) 'how can I help you today?' Meanwhile, the patient feels their precious 10 minutes ticking away. More importantly, the doctor is establishing him- or herself in the role of talker and the patient in the role of listener, which is the opposite of what needs to be happening.

On the subject of introductions, take care over what you call the patient. Don't assume it's OK to call anyone by their first name, not even youngsters or old people, and especially not SCA role-players. Some older people will feel they are being patronised, especially if you use an endearment such as 'sweetheart' or 'darling.' 'Sir' or 'madam' can sound sarcastic. And many young children will be used to being called by a pet name or a shortened form of the name on their records. If in doubt, you could ask, 'What would you like me to call you?' I think it's safest, at least on first acquaintance, to address the patient by title and surname, or given name and family name. If, later in the consultation, as you get to know each other, using the surname starts to feel awkward, you can always ask if it's acceptable to use a first name.

Conversely, some patients may seek to call you by *your* first name, about which you may or may not feel comfortable. What you might regard as overfamiliarity could just be friendliness, but it might equally be an attempt to create a falsely intimate or manipulative relationship. Either way, a discreet way of handling the situation is for you, when addressing the patient, consistently to use their title and surname.

Rapport

The more quickly you can settle the patient into 'telling-you-all-about-it' mode, the better chance you stand of discovering and understanding the full extent of their reasons for consulting you. For this, they need to trust you, to feel comfortable talking to you and to have a sense that you appreciate the significance of what you are being told. In a word, you need rapport. And the best way of establishing rapport is to pay the other person your undivided attention.

This is so important that I'm going to say it again.

The best way of establishing rapport with your patient is to give them your 100% undivided attention − and for them to know *that you are.*

Paying attention

You know from your own experience of family and social life that you can't really understand all the nuances of what someone is telling you if your mind is partly on other things. It's possible to hear every word someone says, yet still miss significant chunks of the information being communicated. To extract the full significance of a patient's narrative, we have not only to listen to their words but also beyond and beneath the words, to what is being hinted at, skirted around, glossed over or omitted. We also have to interpret tone of voice, body language, facial expression and emotional undercurrents. Of course, this is perfectly possible − we've been practising the necessary skills ever since we learned to speak − but it calls for as close to 100% of our attention as we can muster.

You also know from your own experience of conversation that it's not hard to tell whether the person you are talking to is properly attending to what you're saying. If − from the erratic eye contact, the mistiming of their nods and 'uh-huh's, and the irrelevance of their comments − you feel you are not getting the attention you deserve, you feel irritated, rejected, disheartened, resentful, hurt and annoyed. Certainly you feel disinclined to waste any more breath on a narrative that doesn't seem to interest your listener.

It is during the first minute or so of the consultation that the information coming to you from the patient is at its most intense. Don't waste it; it mustn't pass you by because you are not concentrating. Paying your patient your full undivided attention as they begin their story is the single most effective thing you can do to give yourself the best chance of recognising their true agenda. It shows you are concerned and interested, and, knowing this, the patient in turn is encouraged to expand and deepen their opening narrative.

Paying someone 100% attention is hard. For all that you might appear calm on the outside as you greet the patient, on the inside your mind is often noisy with potentially distracting thoughts. Some of them will be medical or work-related; others definitely *not*. There may be some afterthoughts left over from the previous consultation. You might be reminding yourself of something you meant to do during this one, such as check the blood pressure. If it is an SCA station, you'll inevitably feel some anxiety as you prepare to put on a performance that will impress the examiner.

To rein in the wandering mind and concentrate on the patient calls for self-discipline and determination, but it is a skill that can improve with practice. If you are already familiar with a mental technique, such as mindfulness or meditation, so much the better. If not, just telling yourself, *Now concentrate!* as the consultation starts will help.

The computer

There is one potential source of distraction for the doctor (and irritation for the patient) that we must consider explicitly – the computer on your desk.

I am no Luddite; the computer is unarguably an essential tool for clinical and organisational management. But, like any tool, it can be used skilfully or inexpertly, depending on whether *you* control *it* or allow *it* to control *you*. In many ways, the computer affects the consultation like a third person in the room would do. It competes with the patient for your attention and can be as inhibiting to the patient as a mother-in-law on a honeymoon.

Look at it from the patient's point of view. You are about to have a conversation with a relative stranger about matters that might become personal or sensitive. You need to feel that the two of you are in a safe, private space where such confidences are possible. The dimensions of that space are quite precise; it's an ellipse probably no bigger than 100 by 150 centimetres. Having anyone else within this space (including the computer) will feel like a third party intruding into what should be a two-person space. Try this: in your usual consulting room, sit in the patient's chair and see whether the computer is intruding into your personal space. If it is, consider moving it.

If your computer screen is too easily visible to you, you will find the temptation to keep looking at it almost irresistible. You may well justify this by claiming that you need to refresh your memory about the patient's details, past history and medication record, or to see any clinical or Quality and Outcomes Framework (QOF) reminders. My advice (and it is only *my* advice; other views are possible) is that you should check the patient's computer record *beforehand*, but, once the patient is in the room, concentrate on *them*, not the computer, especially at the beginning of the consultation. The conventional wisdom is that, in the name of openness and information-sharing, you should turn the screen so that both you and the patient can see what is on it. I'm not sure I accept this. Most of your patients will be elderly; they will need to use their reading glasses to read the computer screen. But most people don't wear their glasses to consult the doctor. To them, the screen is just a blur, which they know displays information about them, but they can't see what it is. If you have ever found yourself in a similar situation, for instance, when consulting a local government official or a financial adviser, you will know how unsettling this is.

If you really *do* need to access your computer while the patient is talking to you, I suggest that you say, 'Can I just stop you there while I check something on the computer?' The patient will then put their narrative 'on hold,' like pressing the pause button on a video player, and resume where they left off once they know they have your full attention again.

A related question is whether or not you should enter data into the computer in real time while the patient is talking. Again, there is more than one opinion. But mine is that you should not. I hate it when it is done to *me*; it feels rather accusatory, much as I imagine it would feel to be making a statement in a police station. What is more, typing up notes as you go along claims a significant portion of your attention, which I think would be better focused on the patient. Don't flatter yourself that you can multitask; no one can, not really. I'm sure your short-term memory is good enough to remember key features of the consultation until a more suitable moment, such as while the patient is dressing or before you call the next patient.

The consulting room furniture

If you are still in training, you probably don't have much say in how your consulting room is furnished. Nevertheless, the arrangement of the desk and chairs can help or hinder your rapport with the patient, and hence how readily they will open up to you.

It is quite common for there to be one obviously high-status chair in the room – the doctor's. It will probably be leather or smartly upholstered, with castors, a swivel and an adjustable seat. The patient's chair will probably be not so comfortable, maybe a bit shabby, perhaps made of plastic and tubular metal – clearly a lower status chair. The usual justification for this disparity is that the doctor spends long hours seated in the room, whereas the patient is only there for a few minutes, and anyway, you don't want the patient to get so comfortable that they don't want to leave. I don't believe these excuses. The danger is that, even as the patient sits down, their position is being defined by the furniture as inferior to that of the doctor, which subtly suggests that they should only speak when spoken to, as one does in conversation with the monarch. If this is *not* the message you want to convey, then, when you have the option, choose chairs that send a more egalitarian message.

This is particularly important if, as many doctors do, you decorate your room to feel more cosy and personal, perhaps with photographs of your loved ones, pictures or fresh flowers (assuming Health and Safety allow such frivolities). If your consulting room feels too much like your home, the patient will feel like an intruder unless their chair is comfortable enough to suggest they are a welcome guest.

Virtually no one nowadays consults across a desk, doctor on one side and patient on the other. If you do – don't. It is customary for doctor and patient to be separated by just one corner of the desk, perhaps with another chair to one side for anyone accompanying the patient. But even in this more informal arrangement, the distance separating the doctor's and patient's chairs can have an effect on the patient's comfort level. Too far apart, and the patient may feel you don't want to get involved, while too close could be claustrophobic. And patients differ in how much separation they like. What feels comfortable and encouraging for one person may be threatening for another. Age, gender, social and cultural factors all come into play.

If yours is the only chair with castors, it is much easier for *you* to adjust the distance between your chairs than it is for the patient. Most patients, if they feel slightly uncomfortable, will not actually get up, move their chair and sit down again. Instead, they will just take longer to settle down before telling you about their problem. So how can you tell what the 'right' distance is for a particular patient? Only by watching to see whether their body language suggests they're not comfortable and by listening to see whether they embark on their narrative without delay.

Eye contact

As you know from your own social conditioning, eye contact is a very powerful indicator of whether people are in rapport. In a typical one-to-one conversation, most people in the UK probably feel comfortable if eye contact is maintained around 60–70% of the time. Less than this, and we feel the other person is not interested in what we have to say; much more, and we begin to feel intimidated or threatened.

But here again, there can be wide variation between individuals. People who might prefer less than your usual degree of eye contact include: patients who are depressed or embarrassed; some elderly patients brought up to believe 'it's rude to stare'; members of cultures where either the doctor is traditionally seen as an authority figure or where there are strong social norms based on gender or marital status; small children and some teenagers. People who sometimes want *more* intense eye contact than you include: other teenagers; some psychotic patients, especially paranoid schizophrenics, and patients with a manipulative or controlling agenda. Or the patient with the intense gaze may simply be deaf and trying to lip-read.

What is the 'right' amount of eye contact? Whatever amount the patient feels comfortable with; not *you*, the patient.

Body language and facial expression

You don't need me or anyone else to tell you how to interpret people's expressions and body language. Your life experience has given you at least 20 years of practice. But it's surprising how often, in our professional setting, we forget to look pleasant, welcoming and attentive, or to sound interested. If your face, posture and tone of voice show that you are stressed, distracted, irritated, bored or frustrated, you can hardly blame the patient if they don't immediately feel at ease with you.

Figure 4.3 summarises some of the factors contributing to good rapport.

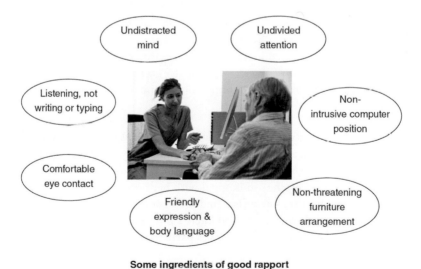

Some ingredients of good rapport

FIGURE 4.3

Starting the Patient's part

Getting the main business of the consultation under way is seldom a problem. You usually only need to say something like, 'How can I help?' or 'What can I do for you?'—and the patient will embark on their story. Indeed, with someone you know well, it may be enough just to smile, say 'Hello,' and wait.

But some patients can be quite unforthcoming at first, seemingly reluctant to tell you much without a good deal of prompting. Such people can be difficult to get into 'telling-you-all-about-it' mode. The consultation might begin with something like this:

Doctor: 'How can I help you?'
Patient: 'It's my knee.' *(Pause)*
Doctor: Tell me about it.'
Patient: 'It hurts.'
Doctor: 'Your knee hurts?'
Patient: 'Yes.'

The temptation now is for you to give up and take the lead yourself, moving straight into doctor-led questioning that really belongs to the Doctor's part. But try to resist this temptation. Stick to your guns and try to find a way of encouraging the patient to tell their story in their own words. Persevere with open questions such as, 'How did it start? How is it affecting you? What do you think might be causing it?' Or just say 'Go on …' with an expectant expression – and wait.

There is a fuller discussion of 'the uncommunicative patient' later in this book in the chapter on 'Some particular challenges.'

Occasionally you will face the opposite problem, the patient who won't stop talking, or whose narrative seems to go round in circles or is full of irrelevant details. A good technique for dealing with this is to give frequent 'mini-summaries,' for example:

Patient: 'I think it was Tuesday, might have been Wednesday. I know it was last week, and it was pouring with rain. Anyway, I was standing there at the bus stop and my knee was that painful. I was going down to see Mother, she's in hospital with her breathing again, I don't know whether you knew that, and she's got arthritis too, and I was thinking, honestly, this blessed knee, I'll have to get something done …'
Doctor: 'So last week your knee was particularly troublesome.'

A mini-summary is a polite way of saying, 'So, to cut a long story short – '
There is more about dealing with an over-talkative patient in the 'Some particular challenges' chapter.

Keeping it going

Once the patient is in narrative 'telling-you-all-about-it' mode, information comes thick and fast. Much of it, obviously, is conveyed through the words the patient uses. You also know that the story is supplemented by *how* it is told – the patient's tone of voice, facial expressions and body language, and the things that are left out or skirted around. In order to understand and interpret all this information, you yourself need to be in full 'listening mode,' with your attention set at maximum. The patient's narrative is often quite tentative at the start of the consultation; if you interrupt, it is easy to knock them back into 'answering questions' mode. But what you are trying to achieve in the Patient's part is to keep the patient doing the telling and you doing the listening. If you start to interrupt too soon or too persistently, you will create the reverse situation, with you asking questions and the patient passively answering them.

Inevitably, as you listen, various doctor-ish thoughts start to come into your mind: possible diagnoses, 'red flag' questions, specific details of the symptoms, etc. But just because a medically relevant question occurs to you, it doesn't mean you have to ask it immediately. This is supposed to be the Patient's part, remember. The time for your medical supplementary questions comes soon, in the Doctor's part, but not yet.

You may also be tempted to take the lead when, as they will from time to time, the patient pauses or hesitates in their narrative, appearing to run out of steam or to be unsure what to say next. But unless you think the patient really *has* run out of things to say, you should resist the temptation and give a gentle nudge, such as 'Please go on,' or 'Can you tell me some more?'

Alternatively, you could try 'echoing' – repeating the patient's last few words in an expectant tone of voice. For example:

Patient: 'My hip's getting worse ...' *(Pause)*
Doctor: 'Your hip?'
Patient: 'Yes. I'm not saying it's *all* the time ...' *(Pause)*
Doctor: 'So it's not troubling you *all* the time?'
Patient: 'No, it's mostly when I go down to make my morning cup of tea. I was thinking about moving into a bungalow, to be nearer my daughter.'

If that doesn't work, you could try some gentle open questions, such as 'How is it affecting you?' or 'Is there anything else worrying you?'

I hope you can hear the difference between the open question 'How is it affecting you?' and the closed question 'How far can you walk?' The patient's reply to the open question will still be *their* story, in *their* words: 'Well, my daughter said she thought I shouldn't be driving.' With this answer, we are still firmly in the Patient's part, getting some insight into the patient's ideas, concerns and expectations. The closed question, clinically relevant though it is, will move the patient out of 'narrative' mode and into 'question-answering' mode, which really belongs in the Doctor's part: 'I don't know, maybe fifty yards? A hundred?'

Probably the only place for closed questions in the early stages of the consultation is when a lack of clarity in the patient's narrative leaves you unsure as to some important fact about the situation they are describing, e.g. 'Is it both knees, or just the one?' or 'When you say it's been for some time, do you mean a few days, or weeks, or several months?'

Here's another challenge for you. Watch the start of two videos of yourself consulting, one that goes reasonably well and another that's not so successful. Make a rough estimate of the relative number of words spoken by you and the patient. I'll wager that in the not so good consultation, it's you who does most of the talking, while in the better one, it's the patient. There's an interesting paradox: at the beginning of the consultation, the less you say, the more you hear. The less you ask, the more you're told. It's very tempting, particularly when you feel under time pressure to get on with the consultation's medical content, to interrupt the patient in the hope of getting them to the point more quickly. The danger is that the point you get them to isn't the real point of the consultation.

Am I suggesting that you should stay silent for the first few minutes of the consultation? No, of course not, not literally silent. For one thing, we all make little murmurs of encouragement – *Mmm*; *uh-huh*; *right, right* and so on – which, together with nods and smiles, reassure the other person that we're listening. But, in the Patient's part, anything you say beyond these verbal punctuation marks should convey only one message – *I really want to understand what you're telling me.* Open questions such as 'What happened next? What else have you noticed? How did it affect you? What did you think was going on? are all fine. So, as I mentioned, are simple closed questions to check matters of fact. So too are comments or remarks such as 'It sounds like that worried you,' 'This isn't anything you've had before, is it?' or 'Remind me who else is at home with you.'

Can you hear the difference between 'It sounds like that worried you' and 'Were you worried this could be cancer?' Or between, 'Has anything like this ever happened before?' and 'What illnesses have you had in the past?' Or between, 'Remind me who else is at home with you' and 'Has anyone in your family had a similar problem?' In each case, the first remark has the effect of encouraging the patient to expand on the story they are *already* telling you and keeps the consultation in the Patient's part. The second is you imposing your own medical agenda, and properly belongs in the Doctor's part.

Give 'receipts' for important points in the patient's story

This is the first time I've used the unexpected word *receipt* in this book, but it won't be the last. In the context of the consultation, a receipt is something you say to the patient that shows you have heard, and understood the importance of, something they have just told you – a kind of verbal 'thank you' note. Let me explain.

As the patient's story unfolds, you get the feeling that some facts or events or details are more significant or noteworthy than others. When you do, it is a good idea to say something that shows the patient that you have noticed the point and have recognised that it is important. Some of the things to acknowledge may seem important to you because of their clinical significance; others may appear important to the patient, even if *you* can't immediately appreciate their relevance.

As an example, let's imagine your patient is David Wren, a man in his early forties. He begins the consultation as follows:

> I'm not one to come to the doctor as a rule, because I know you're busy, but I've been getting indigestion for the last three months. Three months, maybe four … It's just that last night, my wife, the worrier that she is, she showed me this article in a magazine – it was a women's weekly, she's a great reader … It was called "Stomach cancer, the silent killer" …

It's not hard to pick out the significant points in this presentation. I *know you're busy,* probably doesn't matter. *Indigestion for months* does, as does *my wife, the worrier that she is.* The fact that it was a weekly magazine is probably not important, but *stomach cancer, the silent killer,* clearly is. So, if you can do it without interrupting the flow of his narrative, you might punctuate Mr Wren's story as follows:

Patient: 'I'm not one to come to the doctor as a rule, because I know you're busy, but I've been getting indigestion for the last three months. Three months, maybe four …' *(Pause)*

You: 'You've been getting indigestion, you said.'

Patient: 'Yes, I'm pretty sure it's only indigestion. I've just been getting some Rennies from the chemist. It's just that that last night, my wife, the worrier that she is, she showed me this article in a magazine – it was a women's weekly, she's a great reader …' *(Pause)*

You: 'And the article had worried her?'

Patient (with a deep sigh): 'Yes. It was called "Stomach cancer, the silent killer."' *(Pause)*

You: 'Ah, I see. I imagine that got you worried.'

Patient: 'Anyway, I'm sure you'll tell me it's nothing, just indigestion, and I'm being silly, but since she mentioned it, I can't get it out my mind, and I hardly slept …'

Your repetition of the word 'indigestion' during the first brief pause shows Mr Wren that you have picked up his mention of the presenting symptom and helps him begin a story he knows might be difficult. A few moments later, when you say, 'And the article had worried her?' you show you understood that 'worry' is an important feature of what he is telling you. When, after learning what the magazine article was about, you say 'Ah, I see' in a gentle and sympathetic tone of voice, Mr Wren knows you are taking him seriously. 'I imagine that got you worried' confirms that you have grasped just how scared he is and recognised his biggest fear.

These brief remarks that show you've been listening are examples of what I mean by 'receipts.' A paper receipt, such as you might get in a shop, is a confirmation that you have handed over something of value, i.e. money. It's evidence that a transaction has taken place. By the same token, a receipt in this medical context is confirmation – spoken, not written – that the patient has given you something of value, i.e. information, that you have received it, and that you understand its significance.

A receipt, as I am using the term, is quite precise. It clearly refers to a specific detail of what the patient has said: in David Wren's case, the indigestion, the worry, the fear of cancer. A nod, or 'Mmm' or 'Uh-huh' is *not* a receipt; they're not specific enough.

One particularly effective form of receipt is the mini-summary, where, from time to time, you recap the key features of what the patient has been telling you. At this stage in Mr Wren's consultation, for example, you might give him a mini-summary by way of receipt: 'So you've been having what you thought was indigestion, until you and your wife got worried by the article about stomach cancer.'

I'll expand on the usefulness of receipts in the next section of this book and show you how they come into their own when you need to steer the consultation or make transitions from one part to the next. But for now, I just want to encourage you, as you listen to a patient's narrative, to give plenty of receipts; rather more, in fact, than might at first feel natural. Receipts help keep the patient in 'telling-you-all-about-it' mode, and they confirm that you really *are* paying attention and appreciating the implications of what you are being told.

Don't 'medicalise' too soon

A temptation to be resisted is the urge to 'medicalise' the patient's problem too early in their narrative, before you have heard the full story from their point of view and before you have obtained enough information to identify the real problem. In other words, don't jump to premature conclusions. Here's an example of how it's possible to fall into this trap. Remember the patient, a widow in her sixties, who began her narrative as follows:

> I think it was Tuesday, might have been Wednesday. I know it was last week, and it was pouring with rain. Anyway, I was standing there at the bus stop and my knee was that painful. I was going down to see Mother, she's in hospital with her breathing again, I don't know whether you knew that, and she's got arthritis too, and I was thinking, honestly, this blessed knee, I'll have to get something done.

If we're short of time, and particularly if the patient is talkative and we get a bit irritated, a kind of selective aural filter comes into play. We filter out anything that doesn't sound obviously medical, so that what we hear is something like this:

> ###### last week, #### ## ###### ## knee ####### painful ####### arthritis ###### ###### get something done …

Ahah, we think, *osteoarthritis; get an X-ray, prescribe an anti-inflammatory drug, see you in 2 weeks; job done.* But in our hurry to make a medical diagnosis and finish the consultation as quickly as possible, we fail to listen to the totality of what the patient is telling us. And so we miss the fact that the knee pain is only *one* of the patient's concerns; an equally important part of her agenda for this consultation is to arrange some support for when her increasingly dependent mother comes out of hospital.

In this example, it is entirely right that the possible diagnosis of osteo-arthritis should enter our minds. What is *not* helpful is immediately inter-rupting with questions to confirm or refute it. Nor is it helpful to close our minds to other possibilities; nor to assume that just because it happens to be the first thing *we* thought of, it must be the patient's top priority. At this stage of the consultation, the best thing to do is to put the *'arthritis?'* thought on hold – to add it, as it were, to a mental 'to do' list, as something to return to in a few moments when it's our turn to lead the conversation in the Doctor's part.

Don't worry that if you store up the ideas that occur to you during the Patient's part, you might forget them if you leave it until the Doctor's part to mention them. If they are important ideas, you won't forget. Your short-term memory is well up to the task. If you seriously doubt it, you could always write yourself a discreet reminder on a notepad.[1]

Ideas, concerns and expectations (ICE)

The phrase 'ideas, concerns and expectations' was first introduced in 1984 in the classic book *The Consultation: an approach to learning and teaching*, by David Pendleton *et al.*[2] It is now so often quoted in discussing the consultation that it has become something of a cliché. This is a shame: not a shame that it's often discussed, but rather that it has become such a cliché. The fact that it can be abbreviated to the word ICE doesn't help; I've heard doctors, including some experienced GPs who ought to know better, talk about 'icing the patient' or 'doing the ICE.' But behind the cliché is a really important idea – that it helps you deliver good patient-centred care if you have some insight into what the patient thinks is going on, what they're worried about, and how they think you might be able to help.

One unintended consequence of assessing consulting skills in the MRCGP exam has been that some candidates have come to believe that 'doing the ICE' is a formulaic piece of behaviour they have to squeeze into every consultation in order to pass, no matter how clumsily or inappropriately they do it. I once witnessed a GP trainee, just as the consultation was clearly drawing to a close, say, 'Oh by the way, what were your ideas, concerns and expectations?' I could almost hear him thinking, *Phew, I remembered just in time; I hope the examiner noticed.* I *did* notice – but I certainly didn't give him the credit he was expecting. You should want to know how the problem seems from the patient's point of view because you are genuinely interested and curious to understand it, not because you think you'll lose SCA marks if you don't. And you need the information early in the consultation, in time for you to be able to make use of it in your assessment or management plan. Squeezing in some ICE questions at the last minute just shows you don't understand the purpose of them.

Ideas, concerns and expectations form part of the story the patient tells you, or *could* tell you with a bit of encouragement, and therefore ideally belong in the Patient's part. It is best if this information can emerge naturally during the course of the patient's narrative without being forced or obviously fished for. A good way to achieve this is to link your question

---

[1] Assuming you can still use such primitive technology.
[2] Revised version: Pendleton D, Schofield T, Tate P and Havelock P. (2003). *The New Consultation: developing doctor–patient communication*. Oxford: Oxford University Press.

to a receipt for something the patient has already told you. Here are some examples of what I mean.

Doctor: 'This rash you're telling me about (*Receipt*) – did you have any thoughts about what it might be?' (*Ideas*)

Doctor: 'You mentioned your mother had an early menopause (*Receipt*). Were you perhaps thinking your own symptoms could be something similar?' (*Ideas*)

Patient: 'So what with the pain in my knee, and mother being so ill, and her coming home soon, and all the lifting and that ...'

Doctor: 'Yes, you've got a lot on your plate at the moment (*Receipt*). What's the part of it you're most worried about?' (*Concerns*)

Doctor: 'You've mentioned a couple of times that you're sure I'll tell you it's nothing (*Receipt*). Sometimes I find, when people say that, it's because they're afraid it could be something serious.' (*Concerns*)

Doctor: 'It's good that you've been reading about the problem, and looking on the internet (*Receipt*). Did you find anything out about possible treatments?' (*Expectations*)

Patient: 'I know you don't like giving antibiotics if it's just a virus, but I've already had a month off work this year ...'

Doctor: '... so you don't want this to drag on, if there's anything we could do to keep it short.' (*Receipt, confirming expectations*)

In these examples, the doctor is using everyday language, tailored to what has already emerged in the narrative so far. It is important not to sound as if you are just trotting out the same old tired phrases.

Can you see that these ICE questions, even though they are asked by the doctor, are still appropriate for the Patient's part of the consultation? They are designed to help the patient to elaborate on *their* story, not as attempts by the doctor to take over the consultation's direction of travel with his or her own agenda.

You can also see, I hope, how the doctor's enquiries about ICE follow on quite naturally from something the patient has already said, which provides an opening or an opportunity. This technique of acknowledging what the patient tells you and then linking it to a question or statement of your own is an example of what I am going to call 'turning a receipt.' This is an extremely useful technique for steering the consultation (if it needs to be steered), and we will look at it in more detail shortly.

Can you spot what is clumsy or off-putting about the following attempts to find out the patient's ideas, concerns or expectations?

Patient: 'Good morning doctor. I just don't feel well.'
Doctor: 'Why do you think that is?

Patient: 'That's what I've come here to find out!'

Doctor: 'Tell me what you think is causing this.'

Patient: 'You're the doctor; *you* tell *me.*'

Doctor: 'No no, *you* tell *me* …'

Patient: 'I've got this little spot of eczema on my belly, right where the metal stud on my jeans has rubbed it sore.'

Doctor: 'Really? I wonder if you had any thoughts about what it could be.'

Patient: 'I know I should have come earlier, but I've got a constant pain in my stomach, the weight's just dropping off me, and now I've noticed my eyes have gone yellow.'

Doctor: 'What are you worried about?'

Patient: 'I just came in to let you see the new baby, and to thank you for looking after me in the pregnancy.'

Doctor: 'What concerns do you have about him?'

Patient: 'Doctor, I'm so worried about my boy. He just stays in his room all day, and I'm sure he's on drugs, and now he's been suspended from school. I just don't know where to turn.'

Doctor: 'What do you expect me to do about it?'

Patient: 'I won't take up your time, doctor. I just need another month's certificate while my leg is still in plaster.'

Doctor: 'How would you like me to help you with that?'

A note of caution

In 2016, the *British Medical Journal*, in its 'What your patient is thinking' series, published an essay by a patient, Rosamund Snow, entitled '*I never asked to be ICE'd*'.[3] A friend had said to her, after a visit to her GP, 'Don't you hate it when they ask you what *you* think is wrong? I was tempted to say, "Why, don't you know? You're the bloody doctor!"' The author asked her own GP about it and learned that ICE was taught as a communication tool to help get at what patients are worrying about, so that the doctor can deal with those concerns. She happily conceded that 'ICE' questions 'came from good intentions; concerned doctors trying hard to look at the whole patient rather than reduce their patients to a bunch of symptoms.'

> 'I wonder, though,' (the article continued), 'did anyone ask patients how these questions sound or might make them feel? … It either sounds as if they don't know what they are doing or feels like they are testing me, as if they have gathered all the symptoms and know the answer but won't share it. This makes me feel less and less likely to trust that doctor.'

---

[3] Snow R. (2016). I never asked to be ICE'd. BMJ. **354**:i3729.

'A little while later I saw a doctor who I felt had gold standard communication skills. Afterwards I thought about what she had done to make me feel so able to talk to her. Instead of probing my feelings with ICE-based questions, her primary focus was answering the questions I had asked, so I felt she was listening and that we were working together. If she needed information I had not yet volunteered, she made clear why she was asking each question. She shared her thoughts as we went along, so we could discuss them, rather than putting me on the spot – and that made it much easier for me to share my thoughts and worries with her, too. It didn't take long. I had already started to trust her in the first 15 seconds.'

'I understand now why GPs ICE me. But an acronym can't build rapport; it's just another checklist. And it feels like it, on the receiving end.'

In other words, try to understand what your patient thinks and feels about their problem – but don't ICE your patient so obviously that you irritate them. Be sensitive to how different patients might react. Ask ICE-type questions because you genuinely want to know the answers, not just because some pundit or teacher has said you ought to. And explore this territory gently, subtly, imaginatively, and without coming across as mechanical or patronising.

How long should the Patient's part last?

When the composer Mozart asked Emperor Joseph II what he thought of his latest composition, the Emperor said, 'Too many notes, Mozart, too many notes.' Mozart is said to have replied, 'There are just as many notes, Majesty, as are required, neither more nor less.'

Be clear about what needs to happen in the Patient's part. Your aim is to enable the patient to tell you the story they need to tell, neither more nor less. Some stories are simple and short; others are more complicated or sensitive and therefore take longer to tell. In an ideal world, the time available for the Patient's part would be flexible and open-ended. In real life, however, compromises have to be made. You have other patients to see and other responsibilities to attend to. Luckily, it is usually not hard to tell either if you are cutting off someone who still has more to say or if the patient's narrative has largely run out of steam and you can safely move on.

If in everyday practice you regularly catch yourself taking control of the history-taking within the first minute or so, or if your patients quite often seem to want to tell you more about their problem well after you thought the consultation had moved on, you are probably not spending enough time in the Patient's part. If, on the other hand, your consultations frequently over-run and you feel rushed when it comes to decision-making and management-planning, it's possible you might need to be a little more disciplined in how you conduct the Patient's part.

In the SCA, of course, you have 12 minutes for the whole consultation. But this does not mean you should spend exactly 4 minutes in each of the three parts. Ideally, you want to leave at least four or five minutes for the Shared part. It is unlikely that the case scenario will be so simple that the patient can present it in less than two minutes, nor so complicated as to need more than five. Within these broad limits, however, I'm afraid you have to develop your own 'feel' for how to divide your data-gathering time between the Patient's and the Doctor's parts.

A good way of telling whether you have done justice to the Patient's part is to summarise.

Summarise

If after a few minutes, you think you have a good enough understanding of the patient's perception of the problem, you can check by summarising it and seeing if the patient is happy with your summary. Take the earlier example of David Wren and his indigestion.

If you listen attentively and encourage him appropriately with receipts, after a few minutes you could probably say something like: 'So, just to be sure I've understood you correctly – you've been getting what you thought was indigestion for a few months, but your wife showed you an article about stomach cancer, and that has worried you both. But you're otherwise well, apart from work, which can be quite stressful.' If Mr Wren's response is to say, 'That's right, doctor' and to look at you expectantly, then you know you can safely draw a line under the Patient's part and move on to the Doctor's part. But if he says, 'Yes, and cancer runs in the family,' then you know there is a further episode in the patient's narrative – the family history – that you need to hear about.

A summary is, in effect, a comprehensive receipt for everything the patient has so far told you. As the word implies, it should be as concise as possible while still capturing the key features of the patient's narrative. Use the patient's own words wherever you can. 'So Mr Wren, you have a three-month history of dyspepsia and an acute cancer phobia' would *not* be a good summary.

In conclusion

Making a success of the Patient's part is as much about getting your mindset right as about specific consulting skills. The right attitude is 'attentive

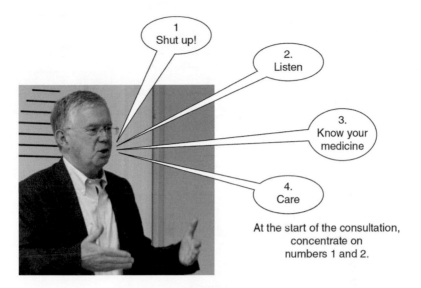

At the start of the consultation,
concentrate on
numbers 1 and 2.

FIGURE 4.4

curiosity' about whatever story the patient chooses to tell you. Try to listen
to it as you would if a close friend was telling you about a new relationship, or if your child was describing a bad day at school. The focus, to start
with, is on the story and the narrator, not on you. David Haslam's *Shut up
and listen!* (Figure 4.4) is good advice. Bite back the medical questions that
will inevitably occur to you; save them up for the Doctor's part, if you can.
Suppress the urge to take over and control the discussion until the patient
really *has* had the time and opportunity to tell their story in their own way.
Don't be in any hurry to think you know what the 'real' problem is; don't
force the patient's problem into a medical diagnosis until you've heard all
the details. Time spent in the Patient's part sometimes feels wasted. But it
seldom is.

All this is counsel of perfection, of course. In real life or in the SCA,
you can't always manage to keep the start of the consultation as patient-
led as I am advocating. Your attention will wander; the patient may need
more prompting than you might like; some medically closed questions will
inevitably creep in; you'll start to worry that time is passing and become
impatient to get on with the medical agenda. But remember, *Perfection is the
enemy of the good.* Just do the best you can.

Figure 4.5 summarises the key ideas for making a success of the Patient's
part. Study it in detail, seeing whether you understand each point. If you're
not sure, go back and re-read the relevant passage.

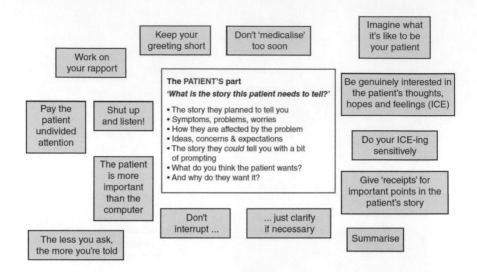

FIGURE 4.5

More about receipts

It was my Danish friend, Dr Jan–Helge Larsen, whom I first heard using the term 'receipt' to describe a little piece of verbal behaviour that effective GPs have been instinctively using for a long time and which can make a powerful contribution to the success of a consultation.

In the previous section, I introduced the idea of a receipt as a way of explicitly recognising key points in the patient's narrative. Think of receipts as doing for a *spoken* narrative what using a highlighter pen does for a *written* text – making the important passages stand out against the background.

We can define a receipt as 'a clear acknowledgment that we have registered, and understood the importance of, what the patient has told us.'

Two parts of this definition need to be emphasised. It needs to be *clear* to the patient that you have understood that what they just told you is *important*. Suppose it's your natural style to nod or grunt, or to murmur 'mmm' or 'right' from time to time while your patient is speaking. (Many of us operate on 'auto-nod' and don't even know that we are making these subliminal encouraging noises. Luckily, the person talking to us usually doesn't notice.) But suppose the patient attaches great importance to what they are telling you. The consultation might begin like this:

Patient: 'I thought I'd best come and see you. I've got a bad knee.'
Doctor: 'Mmm.'
Patient: 'No, it's really painful.'

Doctor: 'Right.'
Patient: 'Believe me, it's absolute agony. Worse than childbirth.'
Doctor: 'Uh-huh.'
Patient: 'I mean, frankly, if something isn't done about it I shall end up throwing myself under a bus.'
Doctor: 'Okay.'
Patient: 'What do you mean, okay? Do you want my death on your conscience?'

The doctor's responses are so non-specific, low-key and uninterested that the patient is forced to 'up the ante' – to give increasingly histrionic accounts of the symptoms – in a desperate attempt to capture the doctor's attention. Instead of a calm, information-rich narrative, we have the makings of a bad-tempered confrontation, which a few simple, well-timed receipts would have prevented.

Patient: 'I thought I'd best come and see you. I've got a bad knee.'
Doctor: 'A bad knee? Okay, tell me about it.'
Patient: 'It's been hurting on and off for ages, but recently it's got a lot worse, especially when I go up and down stairs.'
Doctor: 'So it's affecting your everyday activities now. Did you have any thoughts about what was happening?'
Patient: 'I wondered if I needed an X-ray ...'
Doctor: 'That's certainly a possibility.'
Patient: '... because if it's arthritis, well, I really don't want to have to stop my dancing.'

This exchange takes no longer than the previous dysfunctional one, but it carries us well into the Patient's part of the consultation. We have obtained some relevant clinical information, and already we have some indications of the patient's ideas, concerns and expectations. Let's examine the role receipts have played in this much more successful beginning.

The first receipt is '*A bad knee?*'—Nothing more than a simple repetition of the patient's own words. But, more effective than just '*Mmm,*' it confirms that the doctor is paying attention. The next receipt, '*So it's affecting your everyday activities now,*' shows that the doctor clearly understands the impact the symptoms are having on the patient's life. The third, '*That's certainly a possibility,*' shows the patient that her suggestion of an X-ray is being taken seriously.

Put yourself in the patient's shoes. When the doctor you are talking to makes these brief but perceptive responses, you start to relax. You feel you are in safe hands, knowing that the two of you are on the same wavelength. This encourages you to open up further; you are now firmly in 'telling-the-doctor-all-about-it' mode.

Notice also how the first two receipts – *'A bad knee?'* and *'So it's affecting your everyday activities now'* – were followed by a suggestion from the doctor about how the narrative should continue. *'A bad knee?'* was followed by *'Okay, tell me about it,'* an open-ended invitation to 'tell me what you want me to hear, in your own words.' After *'So it's affecting your everyday activities now,'* the doctor's follow-up question, *'Did you have any thoughts about what was happening?'* gave the patient an opportunity to disclose one of her expectations – *'I wondered if I needed an X-ray.'* These are examples of a technique I call 'turning a receipt' – following up the receipt by giving the consultation a gentle 'steer' as to what happens next. I'll return to this idea shortly. The third receipt – *'That's certainly a possibility'* – was not followed by a steering remark, so the patient continued where she had left off, mentioning her idea (*arthritis*) and concern (*I really don't want to have to stop dancing*).

As well as acknowledging specific details in the patient's narrative – the painful knee, the difficulty with stairs, the possibility of an X-ray – from time to time, you can also use non-specific receipts, such as:

'Thank you, that's really helpful.'
'That's interesting, I'd like to hear more about that.'
'I'm glad you came, so that I can help you with this.'
'You've done the right thing to come and see me.'
'Ah, I see; that makes things clearer for me.'
'Let me just be sure I've understood you correctly' *(followed by a mini-summary)*.

Receipting emotions

Most of the examples of receipts I have given so far have been acknowledgments of factual statements in the patient's narrative. They have referred, for instance, to symptoms (*'I have a rash'*; *'My knee is painful'*; *'I've been getting indigestion'*) or a significant event (*'My wife showed me an article about stomach cancer'*; *'It's worse when I go down stairs'*) or some explicitly stated idea or opinion (*'I was wondering about an X-ray'*; *'I've been reading about it on the internet'*).

But sometimes it can be even more effective to give a receipt for something that *hasn't* been stated in so many words – some unspoken thought, feeling or emotion that you have inferred from the patient's body language, expression or tone of voice. Remember David Wren, the man with indigestion whose wife had been reading about stomach cancer? Suppose he tells you:

'Last night, my wife saw me taking an antacid tablet, and she showed me an article she'd been reading in a magazine about stomach cancer, "the silent killer".'

And then he pauses, his eyes downcast and looking rather pensive.

At this point, you have a range of possible receipts available to you. You could, for instance, say, 'So you're taking antacids.' If you do, Mr Wren will probably continue with, 'Yes, I've been buying them from the chemist; there's a pharmacy just opposite where I work.' Or you could say, 'Your wife showed you a magazine article,' to which he might respond, 'Yes, they've got a new medical correspondent doing a monthly column.' These are both fact-based receipts, and, as you might expect, they are rewarded by an elaboration of the facts – interesting enough, but hardly adding much value to what you know already.

But, being an empathetic doctor, you will sense that beneath Mr Wren's words is an anxiety, so far unspoken, that he might be suffering from something much more serious than he had thought. Suppose you give him a feeling-based receipt for *that* and say:

> 'That must have given you a shock, putting the thought of cancer into your mind.'

Imagine yourself to be Mr Wren, hearing that remark. The doctor has said out loud exactly what you thought and felt but have not yet mentioned. Imagine the relief that now floods through you; this doctor *understands*. You will find it much easier now to talk freely about your anxieties, your ideas, concerns and expectations, your lifestyle, even the state of your marriage. It's likely you'll reply with something like:

> 'Yes, and I haven't stopped thinking about it since. I mean, if, Heaven forbid, it *was* cancer, and I've been ignoring it … You know, I'm still a relatively young man, with a mortgage to pay …'

Receipting a patient's feelings and emotions often has the effect of taking the consultation to a deeper level, where highly significant factors in the patient's story emerge and can be safely discussed. So have the courage, in your own consultations, sometimes to say things like:

> 'That must have worried you.'
> 'I get the feeling you're quite angry.'
> 'I think you're probably quite sad.'
> 'I wonder whether you perhaps blame yourself.'
> 'That sounds really frustrating.'
> 'So the future looks pretty bleak.'
> 'I've known people in a similar situation feel life's not worth living.'

It is important that the words you use in a receipt should match the intensity of the patient's emotion. If a patient is almost apoplectic with rage at having had to wait ten days for an appointment, it will only inflame the situation if you say, 'You seem a bit disappointed with our service.' If, on the other hand, your patient has made an emergency appointment about her child's verruca, for you to say, 'I can see you've been worried sick about this' will just sound sarcastic.

Giving feeling-based receipts may seem something of a risk, carrying the possibility of taking you into emotional territory that may be more difficult to talk about than the superficialities of symptoms and events. 'Why open up a can of worms if you don't have to?' you might ask. To which I'd reply, 'It's more important, and ultimately more efficient, for you to address the problem that matters most to the patient, rather than the one you find most convenient, even if it *is* a bit risky.' The emotional implications of a problem are often at least as important as its factual details. Receipting what you sense to be the truth of the patient's emotions can help them disclose additional layers of relevant psychological information and can strengthen the bond of rapport between you. No risk, no gain.

What and when to receipt

There are no rules, other than that you should consider receipting whatever seems to matter, either to the patient or to you.

In my opinion, we doctors tend to be too sparing with our receipts. For most of us, giving more receipts would probably result in smoother consultations. Try experimenting in your own practice with being more generous with your receipts, and see if it helps things to flow better.

It is certainly possible to overdo receipts. Too many and too frequent can quickly become irritating. The best advice I can give is that you should be guided by your own hunch or instinct. If you are a reasonably sensitive and perceptive doctor, you will already have a feel for what is important in a patient's narrative. As to timing your receipts, there's usually no need to interrupt the patient's flow; the periodic natural pauses in their account will provide plenty of appropriate opportunities.

'Two-part steers'

We use receipts a lot in everyday life, often as the first part of a familiar two-part speech pattern – an observation, followed by a question or a suggestion. The effect is to lead or steer the other person's response in a direction of *our* choosing. Here are some examples from ordinary conversation:

- 'That's a nice shirt. Where did you get it?'
- 'I haven't seen you for ages. How are you?'
- 'It looks like rain, so perhaps you should take an umbrella.'
- 'Jamie, I told you it's supper time. Wash your hands and come to the table.'
- 'You've had that cough for a week now. Maybe you should see the doctor.'
- 'If you're making tea, could I have one too, please?'
- 'You look tired. Let's not go out tonight.'

Now here are some similar two-part steering remarks you might make in a consultation. (We've already seen some examples in the earlier section on ideas, concerns and expectations.)

- 'It's nice to meet you. How can I help?'
- 'We've not met before – tell me a little bit about yourself.'
- 'You mentioned you felt a bit unwell last week. What did you put it down to?'
- 'So the pain came on without any warning. Tell me what happened next.'
- 'I'm not sure I quite understand. Could you give me a bit more detail?'
- 'That sounds unpleasant. But I'm sure we can sort it out.'
- 'I thought you seemed a bit anxious. Is anything worrying you?'
- 'Your certificate is due next week. Are you ready to go back to work?'
- 'OK, you need a further certificate. Is there anything else you'd like to discuss today?'
- 'It doesn't sound like anything serious. But can I just ask, have you brought up any blood?'

The next section takes this idea of the two-part steer a stage further and describes a powerful technique for applying a little leverage to the consultation.

'Two-part steers' in the consultation – turning a receipt

This is a really important section. I'd suggest you don't just read it once and move on; make sure you understand it thoroughly and practise the

79

steering technique I'm about to describe until it becomes a natural part of your consulting style.

When you give a patient receipts for important features in their story, several things result. One is that the patient feels genuinely understood, and this strengthens rapport and encourages the disclosure of further information. Another is that it keeps the patient's story moving forward without unnecessary repetition.

But – and this is the important bit – when you give a clear receipt, something very interesting happens. Just for a moment – one or two seconds at most – the patient will pause and will wait to see whether or not you are going to take over. They will temporarily switch from 'narrative' mode to 'expectancy' mode. If you *don't* follow-up your receipt, after that brief hesitation, they will switch back again, from expectancy back into narrative mode, and will continue where they left off. But if you quickly follow your receipt with a question or suggestion of your own, the patient will accept it and will allow the conversation to turn in the direction you have indicated. It's as if giving a receipt causes a window of opportunity to open where the patient will let you steer the consultation if you wish.

This is so important that I'm going to say it again.

When you give someone a receipt, they briefly pause in mid-narrative and wait for a moment to see if you are going to take over. If you don't, they'll carry on. But if you want to take over, the receipt gives you a window of opportunity to do so.

Imagine this: a friend is telling you about something interesting that recently happened to them. 'I had a great weekend. I went to this concert by a band I hadn't heard before.' If you receipt that remark by saying, 'Sounds like you had a good time,' and you say nothing else, your friend will probably continue, 'Yes, and the best of it was, I got talking with them afterwards and …' The conversation will continue on your friend's territory. But if you say, 'Sounds like you had a good time' (*receipt*) and follow-up with 'That's more than *I* did – my car got a puncture,' your friend will almost certainly ask, 'Oh, what happened?' And the subject of conversation will now switch from the concert to your car problem and its consequences. Control of the topic of discussion has passed from your friend to yourself.

Without the receipt, the conversation will probably go:

Friend: 'I had a great weekend. I went to this concert by a band I hadn't heard before.'

You: 'My car got a puncture.'

Friend: 'Eh? What's *that* got to do with it?'

It will seem to your friend as if you were either not listening or weren't interested in what they were telling you, and they will feel irritated or resentful about your interruption. But if you first give a receipt, it is more likely that the conversation will go like this:

Friend: 'I had a great weekend. I went to this concert by a band I hadn't heard before.'
You: 'Sounds like you had a good time. Which is more than I did. My car got a puncture.'
Friend: 'Oh, bad luck. What happened?'
You: 'I ran over some broken glass. Still, look on the bright side, it got me out of being the designated driver in the evening.'

The receipt helps your friend accept the change of topic without demur; indeed, it will feel as if it follows quite naturally.

I call this two-part sequence – a receipt followed by a steering suggestion of your choosing – 'turning a receipt'. In general terms, turning a receipt – a two-part steer – consists of saying, in effect, 'Thank you for *this*; and now we'll do *that*.'

Let's put this into the context of the consultation. A two-part steer allows you, if you want to, to take the initiative. So if, for whatever reason, you want something different to happen – if, for example, you feel you need to ask a specific question, or change the topic under discussion, or move the consultation on to the next part, or regain control of a consultation that is in danger of becoming dysfunctional – the way to do it is to give the patient a receipt and quickly follow it with your own agenda.

The two-part steer is a powerful and potentially liberating communication skill. Once you've gotten the hang of it, you need never feel helpless or frustrated in a consultation where you know what *needs* to happen but it's just not happening. What you do is, you give the patient a clear receipt, then follow it up with a suggestion that turns the consultation in the direction you think it needs to go.

There are three stages to a successful two-part steer (Figure 4.6). The first is for you to have a clear idea in your mind as to what needs to happen next in the consultation. Then you need to give an effective receipt, i.e. an appreciative acknowledgment of something important the patient has told you. Finally, you follow the receipt by saying something to the patient – the 'steer' – that makes it clear what you want to do or talk about next.

Here are some examples of how a receipt followed by a steer can help at different times in the consultation.

Intention   *To obtain more details about the patient's symptoms*
Receipt: 'Thank you, that's very interesting.'
Steer: 'Please tell me some more about the symptoms you've been getting.'

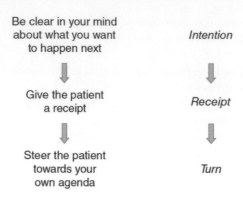

Turning a receipt

FIGURE 4.6

Intention   *To encourage a patient who is reluctant to talk*
Receipt: 'I can see this is a bit difficult for you to talk about …'
Steer: '… but the more you can tell me, the easier it will be for me understand what's worrying you.'
Intention   *To transition to the Doctor's part*
Receipt: 'You've given me a lot of helpful information …'
Steer: '… and now I've got some questions I'd like to ask you.'
Intention   *You want to examine the patient (Doctor's part)*
Receipt: 'I think I've got a clear picture of what's been happening.'
Steer: 'So now I'd like to examine you, please.'
Intention   *To transition to the Shared part*
Receipt: 'Now I've examined you, I think I know what the problem is.'
Steer: 'Let's talk about where we go from here.'
Intention   *To suggest your management plan to the patient (Shared part)*
Receipt: 'I know you've read a lot about this on the internet …'
Steer: '… but first, may I tell you what I'm thinking?'
Intention   *To deal with your own uncertainty*
Receipt: 'I want to be sure you have the best advice…'
Steer: '… so I'd like to get a second opinion from my trainer.'

In these examples, note the general format 'Thank you for *this*; now we'll do *that*.' Also note that the receipts are 'strong' enough to get the patient's attention and thus to open that brief window of expectancy into which you can slip your follow-up steering suggestion. But most importantly, note that you can clearly tell from the words that follow the receipt what it is that the doctor wants to happen next. The receipt acts as a cushion to prevent the doctor's suggestion from appearing too abrupt, but the intention is clear nonetheless.

Using receipts in the Patient's part

Receipts, and using them in two-part steers to bring about a change of direction, can be useful at every stage of the consultation and in many challenging situations. For now, here are some more examples of how this technique can help during the Patient's part, where your aim is to encourage the patient to tell their story in their own words.

Intention *Dealing with a patient who expects you to ask all the questions*
Receipt: 'We haven't met before …'
Steer: '… but I'd like to begin by asking you to tell me as much as you can about why you've come, in your own words.'
Intention *To get a patient who rambles to come to the point*
Receipt: 'There's obviously been a lot happening …'
Steer: '… but perhaps we could focus now on what you think is most important.'
Intention *Dealing with a patient who tells you the same thing over and over*
Receipt: 'I really do understand what you've told me so far …'
Steer: '… but I'm keen to know what happened next.'
Intention *To elicit the patient's ideas (1)*
Receipt: 'This is something you've not had before.'
Steer: 'I wonder what you thought might have caused it.'
Intention *To elicit the patient's ideas (2)*
Receipt: 'You mentioned you'd Googled your condition.'
Steer: 'What did you find out?'
Intention *To find out the patient's concerns (1)*
Receipt: 'You sound quite worried about this.'
Steer: 'Was there anything in particular you were afraid it could be?'
Intention *To find out the patient' concerns (2)*
Receipt: 'This has obviously come as a bit of a shock.'
Steer: 'How do you think it's going to affect you?'
Intention *To discover the patient's expectations (1)*
Receipt: 'There are various ways I could help.'
Steer: 'Did you have any thoughts yourself about what would be best?'
Intention *To discover the patient's expectations (2)*
Receipt: 'I know you're not a great one for taking medication.'
Steer: 'What other kinds of treatment have you heard about?'

Intention *To see whether the patient has any hidden agenda (1)*
Receipt: 'Sometimes when people start by telling me about a relatively minor problem ...'
Steer: '... it can be because they actually have something more serious that's worrying them.'
Intention *To see whether the patient has any hidden agenda (2)*
Receipt: 'You've told me about your acne ...'
Steer: '... but I got the feeling there might be something else on your mind you'd like to discuss.'
Intention *To prioritise the items on a patient's list*
Receipt: 'You mentioned there are several things you wanted to talk about today.'
Steer: 'Shall we start with whatever is worrying you the most.'

Before we leave the subject of receipts for now, I need to clear up a possible misunderstanding. You might think that steering the consultation in the ways I've described in these examples contradicts the principle that, in the Patient's part, you should allow the patient to tell their story in their own words, and not try to impose your own agenda onto the consultation. But the effect of using these receipts is to say to the patient, in effect, 'Tell me more about your problem, or 'Let us see what more you can say with a little encouragement.' As long as the story being told is the problem as experienced from the patient's point of view, and that is the purpose of the receipts you give, then you are still in the Patient's part.

Cues and hidden agenda

Cues and hidden agendas are variations on the theme that patients don't always tell the whole story about why they've come to see you – not at first, anyway, and not unless you help them. A *cue* is something the patient says or does that hints at some important but unexpressed thought or feeling. *Hidden agenda* is something the patient wants from the consultation but which, for conscious or unconscious reasons, they don't explicitly mention.

If you're an SCA candidate, let me tell you something a cue is *not*. It is *not* a tiny piece of information crucial to the case but so heavily disguised that you'll probably miss it and thereby fail the station. The examiners are not so devious.

And if you're a practising GP, let me reassure you about something that hidden agenda is not. Hidden agenda is *not* a time-wasting distraction used by a troublesome patient to make your already busy day even busier. Patients are not so spiteful.

So why don't patients simply come straight out with whatever it is they want from you? Because they're humans, that's why. Because they sometimes feel insecure, awkward, scared, muddled, nervous, embarrassed or ashamed. Because they have needs and motivations that operate below the threshold of conscious awareness. Because they often lack the vocabulary to express difficult thoughts and feelings. Because, in short, they are much like the rest of us.

OK, you might grudgingly protest, *but if a patient can't, or won't, be bothered to say what's on their mind, it can't be all that important, can it?* If only that were true. If only a problem ignored or a problem denied were a problem resolved. A patient's deep-seated anxieties won't go away just because a stressed or overworked doctor turns a blind eye on them. They will persist and resurface, and find other ways of expressing themselves until someone – and why should it not be you? – recognises and addresses them. And anyway, do you really want to be a doctor who only deals with superficialities? Do you really want to spend your career acting as if people had only surfaces and no depths? However attractive that approach may seem when you're having a bad day, in the long run, it is a sure route to disillusionment and burnout. There is a pride and a satisfaction to be found in searching with a patient for the origin of their distress, facing it with them, and together finding a way back to peace of mind.

Cues

Cues to a patient's underlying concerns can be behavioural, verbal or non-verbal.

The way a patient behaves or sets up the consultation can send powerful symbolic signals. If a husband and wife attend together to discuss the failing health of an elderly relative, particularly if one of them has taken a day off work to keep the appointment, you can be sure they intend their 'something must be done' message to be taken seriously. The mother who sits to one side with arms folded and a face like thunder while her 15-year-old daughter tells you she has missed three periods, is showing you very clearly what she thinks of the situation. The infrequent attender who starts to make weekly appointments about minor illnesses is trying to tell you something, even if you don't yet know what it is.

Non-verbal cues are communicated through facial expression, body language, tone of voice, eye contact and so on. We are all familiar with the hesitant speech of someone who is nervous; the avoidance of eye contact that suggests embarrassment; the way anxiety is revealed in physical restlessness; the moistening eye of someone on the verge of tears. You don't need me or anyone else to teach you to interpret these signs; you already have decades of experience of 'reading' people in your own family and personal life.

Probably the majority of significant cues in consultations are verbal – the things your patient says or *doesn't* say. Reading between the lines of the following remarks, what underlying issues do you think might be being implied?

- 'You'll probably tell me, I'm sure you'll tell me, I'm just wasting your time.'
- 'Honestly, that boy of mine, he's just like his father.'
- 'They do say a drop of red wine does you good, don't they?'
- 'My wife? Well, we're not still teenagers, and of course, she gets very tired.'
- 'I expect I just need a tonic.'
- 'My word, you don't look old enough to be a doctor.'
- 'Everything's fine at home – we've got a nice house, no money worries, and the children are no trouble.'

Remarks like these clearly have a subtext, and one that's quite likely to be relevant to the problem being presented. Here again, you can probably rely on your own life experience to supply the right interpretation – but only if you notice the cue in the first place. The best way to give yourself the best chance of picking up such potentially important nuances in the patient's story is to pay it your very best attention during the Patient's part.

Responding to cues

What should you do when you pick up a cue? Sometimes – nothing. Not every glimpse of a patient's unexpressed thoughts needs to be acted on. If you were to pounce every time the patient twitches or hesitates, the consultation would quickly become intolerable. Only *you* can judge whether the information you think you might obtain is worth interrupting the patient's narrative for. Sometimes the patient, knowing that some significant topic is being hinted at, will pause and look expectantly at you, as if to say *I'm giving you the chance to follow it up; please take it.*

If you're not sure or if you feel you don't want to interrupt, you can always defer clarifying a cue until later in the consultation and add it to your mental 'to do' list for the Doctor's part. But if you *do* decide to follow-up on what you think might be an important cue, how can you do it? In the same way I described earlier for taking temporary control of the consultation – by turning a receipt. You acknowledge what you've understood from the patient and follow it with an indication of what you'd like to know next.

Many cues lend themselves to a two–part 'steering' response. Here are some suggestions for applying this technique to the examples I gave earlier:

Cue: 'You'll probably tell me, I'm *sure* you'll tell me, I'm just wasting your time.'

Response: 'I'm sure you're not. But you sound worried …'

Cue: 'Honestly, that boy of mine, he's just like his father.'

Response: 'Is he? Tell me about his father.'

Cue: 'They do say a drop of red wine does you good, don't they?'

Response: 'So some people say. How much is a "drop" in your case?'

Cue: 'My wife? Well, we're not still teenagers, and of course, she gets very tired.'

Response: 'Does she? And is that affecting your relationship?'

Cue: 'I expect I just need a tonic.'

Response: 'Possibly. Is life pretty hard at the moment?'

Cue: 'My word, you don't look old enough to be a doctor.'

Response: 'I'll take that as a compliment. Why don't you put it to the test, and tell me how I can help you?'

Cue: 'Everything's fine at home – we've got a nice house, no money worries, and the children are no trouble.'

Response: 'Excellent. But you didn't mention your husband. Everything fine with him as well?'

Hidden agenda

Much of what I've said about cues also applies to hidden agendas. You can often detect that the patient wants more from the consultation than they initially tell you by watching and listening carefully at the beginning. If you get this impression, you have to make a judgement call as to whether to comment on it at the time, defer commenting until later or keep your thoughts to yourself.

But if the supposed hidden agenda has implications for how the present consultation needs to be conducted, the earlier you address it, the better. For example, a consultation might begin:

You: 'How can I help today?'

Patient: 'How long have you got? My knee, for a start.'

Immediately, you suspect this patient has a list of problems. It is helpful for you to know at the outset what else is on the list, rather than have further items produced every few minutes. Here again, the trusty two-part receipt can come to your aid. You reply:

> It sounds as if you've got several things to discuss. Tell me what else is on your list, so that I can plan how best to use our time.

Here are some further examples of remarks that suggest the patient may have a hidden agenda. What do you think it might be? And how do you think you might respond, if at all?

* 'Of course, I normally see Doctor X about my tiredness. But I thought I'd come and see *you* this time, get another opinion.'
* 'I hope you don't mind, but I was making cakes and I thought you might like some.'
* 'Hi Doc. My name's John, but my friends call me Jonjo.'
* 'Do you have any children of your own, Doctor?'
* 'It's three months now since my accident, and the pain from my whiplash injury isn't getting any better. I want you to make a note of that in my records.'

Health beliefs

As well as their thoughts about a particular problem, patients – people – have more general health beliefs about how their bodies work, what can go wrong with them, and how they should be treated. As doctors, we would prefer health beliefs to be based on factual knowledge interpreted within a logical and scientific framework. But many patients have health beliefs that are less than completely rational. Their knowledge of anatomy and physiology may be sketchy. They may gain most of their views about disease and its treatment from family members, the media or Doctor Google. They can be influenced by fads and fashion. They may have irrational trust in, or suspicion of, the medical profession. Some patients may be unshakeably wedded to theories of disease and alternative forms of therapy which we discredit.

The effect of patients' health beliefs is most apparent during the final Shared part of the consultation, when a management plan acceptable to both doctor and patient is being negotiated. If the doctor's explanation and proposals conflict with the patient's health beliefs, it becomes much more difficult to reach agreement. Every GP has experienced the frustration of trying to achieve a compromise with a patient who is convinced that 'antibiotics cure all infections,' or who 'doesn't believe in drugs,' or thinks that 'a scan will give us the answer,' or is sure that they will only get the best treatment if they see a specialist privately.

If a patient has health beliefs potentially conflicting with your own, the earlier in the consultation you can discover them, the better. Doing so enables you to spot potential disagreements in advance and to tread cautiously. However, with a topic so rich in individual variation, it is not possible to identify health beliefs by systematically asking standardised questions. Instead, you may have to rely on picking up subtle indications – reading between the lines – during the Patient's part. In the next three examples, the patient's health beliefs can be clearly discerned, and may well affect later discussion in the Shared part of the consultation.

- 'I know technically I'm overweight, but we're all big-boned in my family.' *(The patient is in denial and unwilling to take any responsibility for her obesity.)*
- 'I've tried everything – arnica, Reiki, acupuncture …' *(The patient makes indiscriminate use of alternative therapies, and may be reluctant to accept orthodox medical treatments.)*
- 'I'm not going to tell you how much I drink. I don't think that's anyone's business but my own.' *(The patient probably drinks to excess, but doesn't want to face the fact.)*

Yet again, it's a matter for your own judgement as to whether to challenge what the patient has said. In these examples, it might be best merely to make a mental note of it. If you *do* decide to respond, turning a receipt can help you do so without too much risk of provoking a confrontation. So you might say:

- *(to the big-boned patient)* 'That certainly puts you at a disadvantage; but it's still possible to keep your weight within healthy limits.'
- *(to the alternative therapy enthusiast)* 'I admire you for trying to sort things out yourself. I hope that doesn't mean you won't let me try to help in *my* way.'
- *(to the secret drinker)* 'Absolutely. And I wouldn't ask if it wasn't relevant to your health.'

But in these next examples, the patient appears to be under a misapprehension that, if not addressed, could lead to a seriously dysfunctional consultation.

- 'I'm afraid I have a complaint. You saw my 16-year-old by herself yesterday, and I should have been notified.' *(The patient is wrongly informed about confidentiality.)*

- 'I know you get paid extra if you don't refer me to hospital.' *(The patient mistrusts the motives behind your recommendations.)*
- 'I read this article that proves vaccines cause brain damage.' *(You and the patient have different views about the nature of reliable evidence.)*

Think what you might say in reply to each in order to try and close the gap between your and the patient's perception of the situation. As you know, the general format for turning a receipt is:

'You mentioned …' or 'I noticed …,' followed by 'I suggest …'

How about:

- *(to the angry parent)* 'I can see you're upset. Perhaps I should explain about young people's right to confidentiality.'
- *(to 'You get paid extra')* 'That's an interesting idea. But it's actually not true.'
- *(to the vaccine doubter)* 'Yes, there's been a lot about it in the media. But much of what you read is dangerously misleading.'

Cues and hidden agenda in the SCA

As I hinted at the start of this section, there is a widely-held but erroneous belief that SCA cases are littered with cues and hidden agendas of immense subtlety but vital importance, cunningly concealed by the examiners in order to trick candidates into missing the whole point of the station. This is a myth; please do not believe it. More importantly, do not conduct your SCA consultations as if it were true. Every SCA case is designed to be as realistic as possible, and the role-players are trained to speak and behave as an ordinary person would during the consultation as it unfolds. This means that any cues to issues beneath the surface will be no less obvious than they are in real life. There is no need to read any more into a role-player's performance than you would back home in your own practice with a real patient. If a patient – real *or* simulated – says to you, 'My mother had a terrible time with *her* change of life,' I'm sure you would recognise this as a cue to ask the patient what she feels about her own approaching menopause. Don't, through paranoia, allow yourself to be side-tracked into fruitless pursuit of hypothetical secrets, as in the following exchange (and I exaggerate to make the point):

Patient: 'I don't seem to be sleeping very well these days.'
You: 'I notice you looked away when you told me that. Is there any sexual abuse going on? Or drug addiction? Do you have any suicidal thoughts?'

A former teacher of mine used to call this 'bucketing an empty well.' It wastes time, irritates the role-player and causes you unnecessary anxiety. If it's not too much of a paradox to say so, in the SCA, you can take the cues at face value.

Transitioning from the Patient's part to the Doctor's part

So far, in the Patient's part, you have concentrated on understanding the problem from *the patient's* perspective, getting *the patient's* opinion of what is important, and *the patient's* thoughts about what might be going on. Most of what you have said and done has been with the intention of helping the patient give you as comprehensive an account as possible of the situation from their point of view. But the patient's version is only part of the story. Understanding the problem in the patient's terms is all very well – indeed, it's essential – but it's not enough. If the patient is to benefit from your medical expertise, you have to translate or reframe it into medical terms, into something you as a doctor can work with. You have to take a problem that to the patient seems puzzling or worrying, and try to understand it in a way that makes medical sense to you. You have to sift out the relevant features of the patient's narrative and supplement them with whatever additional information you need to bring the problem within reach of your medical knowledge and resources. Figure 4.7 illustrates the shift from Patient's part to Doctor's part.

This harvesting of additional medically relevant information is going to occupy the Doctor's part. But for this to happen, both you and the patient have to change what you have been doing so far. *You* have to stop being a listener and facilitator and instead take the lead in data-gathering. And the patient has to reciprocate by switching from narrative 'telling-the-doctor-all-about-it' mode into 'answering questions' mode.

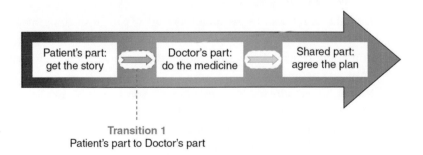

Transition 1
Patient's part to Doctor's part

FIGURE 4.7

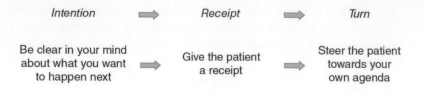

FIGURE 4.8

How is this shift to be achieved? With a two-part steer. You turn a receipt. You acknowledge what has gone before, then indicate what is to happen next. In effect, you say, *'I understand what you've told me so far; now I'd like to ask you some questions of my own.'*

Remember the three stages of turning a receipt (Figure 4.8)?

Let's think about each stage in order and how they can be applied to transitioning to the Doctor's part, beginning with 'being clear about what you want to happen next.'

If you have followed the suggestions I have given you about conducting the Patient's part, you will have encouraged the patient to tell you as full a story as possible, resisting the temptation to interrupt other than to make sure you fully understand what you are being told. You will have managed not to ask your medical questions as soon as you think of them and tried not to 'medicalise' the patient's problem prematurely. Instead, you will have been storing up – as it were, in your mind's 'memory cache' – a 'to do' list of points you want to clarify and further information you need to obtain. For instance:

- You might want to fill in some further details of the patient's history – the symptoms, their timing and their consequences.
- If some parts of the patient's story have been vague or ambiguous, you may wish to clarify them.
- It might be relevant to ask about any other past or ongoing medical problems.
- You might want to know more about the patient's psychological state or social circumstances.
- If they haven't already been mentioned, you may wish to check the patient's ideas, concerns or expectations.
- You may have picked up some cues that the patient has hidden or additional agenda that has not so far emerged.
- If it is clinically relevant, there could be 'red flag' questions you need to ask.

- Again, if it's clinically relevant, you may need to perform a physical examination.
- Particularly in an SCA case, you might want to reassure yourself that you've not missed the point and that there isn't some important aspect of the case that you have completely overlooked.

You may be afraid you won't remember everything you want to ask about in the Doctor's part, and will be tempted therefore to ask your doctor-centred questions as soon as you think of them during the Patient's part. To reassure you, I would say this: firstly, the sky will not fall if you *do* sometimes interrupt the patient's narrative with a Doctor's part question. Just try not to do it too often. Try to preserve as much of a patient-centred focus as possible during the early stages of the consultation, and as far as possible, keep the patient in narrative mode. Secondly, if the points you want to raise in the Doctor's part are important, you *won't* forget them; your brain is cleverer than that. Thirdly, if you really *do* have a poor memory, it is OK during the Patient's part unobtrusively to make notes of things you want to come back to.

Turning now to the 'giving the patient a receipt' part of the transition: the single most useful and effective way of doing this is to summarise – to offer the patient a condensed version of what you have understood to be the key features of the patient's narrative and see whether the patient agrees with your summary.

Summarising as a transition

A summary is an all-inclusive receipt for everything the patient has so far told you during the Patient's part. As with any receipt, the patient will pause and listen, and if you don't follow it up (or if they feel you've left out something important), they will then continue with what they were telling you before. But if you follow your summary with an indication of what you want to happen next (which is now to move on to the Doctor's part), the patient is likely to accept your suggestion. And most importantly, from the patient's point of view, moving on will feel like the logical next stage in the consultation. Your questions will seem to follow quite naturally from what has gone before.

What makes a 'good' summary?

- A good summary is well-timed. It should come when the patient's narrative seems to be running out of momentum, or when you think you have understood its main points. If you are lucky, on a good day, these two will coincide. If you summarise too soon, perhaps because you have a tendency to 'premature medicalisation,' you might miss significant additional information which the patient is inhibited from telling you. On the other hand, if you are too afraid of missing something important or if you are nervous about taking control of the consultation process, you may leave summarising too late and waste valuable time.

- A good summary is 'signposted,' so that the patient knows what is coming. You might, for example, say, 'Just so that I can be sure I've got things clear in my mind, what you've told me is …' or, 'Let me check that I've got this right.' Don't always use the same words for every patient; otherwise, you will start to sound like a robot.

- A good summary is just that – a summary. It concisely restates the main points of what the patient has told you and leaves out things that don't seem to matter to you or the patient. A good summary does *not* begin, 'It might have been Tuesday or maybe Wednesday, and you were standing at the bus stop in the rain.'

- A good summary recapitulates not only the facts revealed in the patient's story but also what you have learned about the patient's interpretation of them. You might want to mention the patient's feelings, such as anxiety or sadness, and also perhaps their ideas, concerns and expectations. This would be a good summary: 'You've come today because your knee pain is getting worse, and you're worried it's going to affect how you can look after your mum when she comes out of hospital.'

- A good summary uses the patient's language, not yours. This would *not* be a good summary: 'You've attended today because your query osteoarthritis is potentially impacting on your role as primary carer for your mother.'

- No matter how good your summary is, there is always the possibility that the patient will want to add something to it or correct something they think you may have misunderstood. So, if you are a good summariser, you will watch and listen carefully to how your patient responds to your summary, so that you can modify it if necessary.

- A good summary, confirmed by the patient, sets your *own* mind at rest, reassuring you that it is safe to proceed to the Doctor's part. If you are not sure that you have really understood the patient's agenda, or if you have a lurking suspicion that you might have missed something really important (a common anxiety in the SCA), it is perfectly acceptable at this stage for you to ask, 'Is there anything else you'd like to tell me?' or, 'Have I missed anything that's important for me to know about?'

Transitioning without a summary

Not every consultation needs a summary to make the transition from Patient's to Doctor's part. Remember the big picture; the point of your data-gathering is to identify the right problem, i.e. to understand what this particular patient needs from the consultation. You are doing this by, first of all, getting the patient's account of the problem clear in your mind, and then supplementing it with whatever medically relevant information you need. It may be that the patient's agenda is so obvious or so straightforward that no summary is needed, and you can go ahead with your doctor-led questions without further ado. For example, a patient might say, 'As you see, doctor, I've still got my leg in plaster, so I just need a certificate for another month.' There is no point in trying to summarise this request; indeed, it would be hard to do so, and you would sound foolish if you tried.

Another instance where a formal summary might be inappropriate is when the patient has come to tell you about an emotionally fraught situation, such as a broken marriage, or a delinquent child, or the death of a parent. In such cases, the story usually emerges gradually from exchanges and interactions between patient and doctor; the distinction between Patient's and Doctor's part is less clear-cut. Any summary might best be deferred until just before you are ready to move on to the Shared 'what-shall-we-do-about-it?' part of the consultation.

Introducing the Doctor's part

The final stage in turning a receipt is steering the patient towards your own agenda. You should, by now, have a pretty clear idea of what questions you want to ask, or what further information you want, or what issues you want to discuss further. So, depending on your agenda, after your summary you might say:

- 'There are some medical questions I'd like to ask you now.'
- 'I'd like to get a few more details about your symptoms.'
- 'I'm not quite clear about …'
- 'Could you tell me how all this has made you feel?'
- 'I don't know much about your situation. Who else is there at home?'
- 'I need to ask some questions just to rule out anything serious.'
- 'I'm not sure what it is that's worrying you most.'
- 'I'm not sure how you would best like me to help you.'
- 'I noticed you mentioned your husband likes a drink. Is that a bit of an issue, perhaps?'
- 'I get the feeling there might be something else on your mind.'

- 'Was there anything else you wanted to discuss today?'
- 'Is there anything else you haven't mentioned that you think it would be helpful for me to know?'
- 'I'd like to examine you now, if I may, please.'

'Turning' remarks like these show the patient that you are taking over the questioning, and give a useful indication of what to expect next. And now you are ready to proceed with the doctor-led information-gathering part of the consultation.

There will usually be quite a few questions or topics you want to explore during the Doctor's part. But you don't need to flag them all up at once. If (in the case of David Wren) you were to say, 'I want to ask you more about the indigestion, and whether you've lost any weight, and what you thought it might be, and if your wife is worried, and whether you smoke, and also I need to examine you,' both you and the patient will be hopelessly confused. To launch the Doctor's part, a single enquiry is enough – perhaps the one you think is most important or the one that seems to follow most naturally from the end of the Patient's part. This will be enough to 'flip' the patient out of narrative mode and into 'question-answering' mode, which is all you are trying to achieve at this point.

Making a success of the Doctor's part

You will probably breathe a sigh of relief as you reach the Doctor's part of the consultation (see Figure 4.9). Here you are on familiar ground; how to take a doctor-centred history was, after all, drummed into you at medical school, and it remains the default approach most of us tend to revert to under pressure. Ironically, however, its very familiarity poses a potential danger. All your training before you entered general practice stressed the importance of making a diagnosis before proceeding to treatment. What's

The DOCTOR'S part
'What more do I need to know?'

- Clarification of the symptoms/problem
- Other medically-relevant questions
- 'Red flag' questions
- Exploration of cues or hidden agenda
- Ideas, concerns & expectations
- Physical examination, if indicated
- Diagnosis, differential diagnosis or 'working assessment'
- Summarise

FIGURE 4.9

more, hospital-based medicine has a very clear idea of what a diagnosis *is* – it's an explanation of a patient's symptoms in biological terms. The danger is that, in the Doctor's part of a general practice consultation, you might be tempted to pursue a physical diagnosis to the exclusion of everything else. But as you know, in general practice, we are trying to achieve a more comprehensive insight into a patient's problem, one which extends beyond a purely physical diagnosis (if there is one) and can include psychological, emotional, family, social, economic, ethical and cultural factors as well.

That said, if you're an SCA candidate, and even though the C in SCA stands for 'consultation', and even though your knowledge base is tested elsewhere in the MRCGP, it is nonetheless very important to have an up-to-date working knowledge of everyday clinical medicine. Remember David Haslam's dictum – after 'shut up' and 'listen' comes 'know your medicine.' You can't bluff your way through the SCA with a bravura display of niceness and communication skills. No patient ever died because the doctor neglected to elicit their expectations, but overlooking the early signs of pancreatic cancer, or not knowing how to manage a wheezy child, or underestimating the depth of a patient's depression can be catastrophic.

The single most common reason for underperforming in the SCA is failing to make a satisfactory management plan. Often, this is the result of running out of time. But, regrettably, it can sometimes reflect an inadequate knowledge of current best practice in clinical scenarios that, frankly, should be within the competence of every practising GP. The clinical knowledge required to pass the SCA is what can be reasonably expected of you in order to keep your patients safe – no more, but certainly no less. So however else you prepare for the exam, I would urge you to see lots of patients, read the journals and reflect regularly on the quality of your clinical decision-making.

Phew! Lecture over. Now let's think about what needs to happen in the Doctor's part if you are to achieve its aim of completing the data-gathering phase of the consultation. We'll start by reviewing some of the categories of information you might need to enquire about. After that, we'll look at some of the tactics you might use to make this part of the consultation as productive as possible.

Things you might include in the Doctor's part

Clarifying the details of the patient's presenting problem

Your knowledge of medicine will suggest to you what further details you need, in addition to whatever the patient has already told you, in order

97

to make a diagnosis or a differential diagnosis, or to achieve a workable understanding of the patient's reason for attending. If the problem is a clinical one, these might include the timing, sequencing and evolution of symptoms and their impact on the patient's life. Now is also your chance to clarify any uncertainties or ambiguities in the patient's narrative if you feel it is necessary for your understanding.

'Red flags'

For some clinical presentations, there will be 'red flag' symptoms you need to ask about in order to detect or exclude serious or urgent problems. Keeping your patients safe is a fundamental principle of primary care and is explicitly included in practically every SCA case-marking schedule.

Other medically relevant information

You may, for example, want to enquire about

- past medical history,
- past and current medication,
- allergies,
- family history,
- other continuing or chronic medical conditions.

There may also be some QOF-related prompts or reminders on the computer or in the notes, which you might feel it is important to ask about. (We'll look at how to deal with doctor-led agenda shortly.) The key thing here is 'relevance'; asking a patient who has just found a lump in her breast when she last had a tetanus booster would be irrelevant and insensitive, as well as wasting precious time.

Psychosocial factors

As a GP, you know that numerous non-physical factors contribute to, and are affected by, the patient's biomedical problem. These include:

- mood and emotional state, such as anxiety or depression;
- possible cognitive impairment, thought disorder or memory failure;
- personality, e.g. optimistic, pessimistic, fatalistic, passive, assertive;
- family circumstances;
- significant relationships, including friends and social support network;
- ethnicity, cultural background or religion;
- sexual orientation;
- financial circumstances;

- employment status;
- lifestyle (including, but not confined to, smoking, alcohol, recreational drug use, diet, exercise and sport);
- ambitions, hopes, plans and life priorities.

If time were unlimited, it might be interesting to explore all or most of these considerations with every patient. But in reality, you have to make a judgement as to what psychosocial factors might be relevant in the particular case, and to be selective in choosing what to explore and in how much depth. This selectivity cannot be taught; your best guide will be your own personal experience of what things are important in life. If you can, talk to the patient much as you would a friend or family member, trusting your instincts to sniff out the things that are likely to matter in the context of the presenting problem.

Ideas, concerns and expectations (ICE)

The essence of the three-part approach to the consultation is that you start by trying to understand the problem from the patient's point of view before moving on to see it in medical terms. Ideally, therefore, you should encourage the patient to tell you during the *Patient's* part what they think is going on (ideas), what are their chief worries (concerns), and how they would like you to help (expectations). But if these considerations have not emerged during the Patient's part, and if you think they might be important, you have another opportunity to explore them now, during the Doctor's part.

It often happens that a patient's ideas, concerns or expectations are either perfectly obvious or can be reasonably inferred without your having to spell them out. If, for example, a heavy smoker tells you he is coughing up blood, which was what his own father did before he was diagnosed with lung cancer, it would be extremely insensitive for you to ask him what he is worried about and what he wants you to do about it. But, understandably, if this was an SCA case, you would not want the examiner to think you had neglected to explore these important matters. In such a situation, you might try this: rather than ask questions, you could give the patient a brief summary of what you think he is thinking. Say, for instance, 'So naturally you're worried you might have the same condition as your father, and you're hoping I can put your mind at rest.' For you to give voice to your patient's unspoken thoughts like this avoids asking unnecessarily obvious questions and demonstrates your empathy to both patient and examiner.

Cues, hidden agenda and health beliefs

We looked in detail at how unspoken thoughts are communicated when considering the Patient's part, because that's where they are most often spotted. You may well have picked up some cues and explored them at the time. But if not, you have a further opportunity to do so, should you choose, in the Doctor's part. It may be that the moment has passed; use your discretion as to whether or not probing the patient's unstated concerns helps you achieve the overall aim of your data-gathering, which is to identify the chief problem that needs your attention. If you *do* decide to do so, a useful form of words is something like: 'I remember earlier you told me … and I'm wondering whether …'

Explain why you're asking ('Signposting')

When you ask your questions in the Doctor's part, it often helps if the patient knows *why* you're asking them. You yourself know the reasons, but the patient may not, and the uncertainty can make them guarded in their response. Or they may try to guess what you're thinking and often guess wrongly. For instance, if, suspecting hyperthyroidism, you ask the patient whether they have lost any weight, the patient may construe this as meaning you think they have cancer and start to panic. But if you preface your question with a brief explanation – 'I'm wondering whether you might have a thyroid problem, which could make you lose weight' – the patient (or the SCA examiner) will know what you are doing, and will also be reassured that *you* know what you are doing. Here are some other examples of this technique, which is often referred to as 'signposting':

- 'There are a few questions I need to ask to make sure this isn't anything too serious.'
- 'I'd like to ask you a bit more about the pain.'
- 'This may sound an odd question, but it's to find out if you've had any internal bleeding. Have you ever passed any motions that looked rather like road tar?'
- 'When someone's depressed, it's important for me to ask whether they've ever felt life wasn't worth living.'

Don't overdo your signposting; often the reason for your question is obvious. But if you think it might be unexpected or unsettling, then tell the patient why you're asking.

Sequencing your questions

As a general principle, it is best if your questions in the Doctor's part move from the general to the particular. Try starting by giving the patient a prompt as to the topic you would like to know more about. Then let them tell you about it in their own words – much as you did in the Patient's part, the difference being that now it is you choosing the topic. So you might say, 'Tell me what you know about eczema,' or 'Could you tell me a bit about your family?' or 'Remind me what tests you've had done in the past,' or 'I see from your notes you've seen several other doctors about this problem,' or 'I'm not quite clear what it was that made you decide to come and see me.'

You probably know the difference between 'open' and 'closed' questions. Open questions allow the patient unlimited choice about how they will reply. There is no restriction on the range of possible answers. Examples are: 'How did it start?'; 'What happened next?'; 'How did that make you feel?'; 'Why do you think that?'; 'What did you think it was?'; 'What's been happening at work?' Open questions keep the patient in 'telling' mode and encourage them to keep disclosing fresh information. If this is what you want to achieve, persevering with open questions is a good way of making it happen.

Closed questions, on the other hand, have only a limited number of possible answers, often either 'Yes' or 'No,' or 'Don't know.' Examples are: 'Have you had any vomiting?'; 'Where was the pain?'; 'Was it constant, or did it vary?'; 'How much weight have you lost?'; 'When did we last check your blood pressure?'; 'Do you smoke?' Once you start to ask closed questions, the patient quickly comes to expect more of the same and settles firmly into 'question–answering' mode. If this is what you want to happen – for instance if the patient is unhelpfully talkative – asking closed questions will usually have the desired effect.

'Indirect' questions, grammatically speaking, are not questions, in that they don't have a question mark at the end of the sentence. They are statements or suggestions that *imply* a question, and to which the patient will respond as if they had been asked a question, e.g. 'Most people find it a bit awkward to talk about sex,' or 'There's been a lot in the papers about depression,' or 'I imagine life is pretty stressful sometimes,' or 'That must have been upsetting.' Indirect questions are particularly helpful for raising and exploring subjects that the patient might find painful or embarrassing.

It's important in the Doctor's part to keep your mind as open as possible for as long as possible. So it is probably good tactics in the early stages of the Doctor's part to use mainly narrative prompts, open questions and indirect questions, and to save closed questions for later, for dotting the 'i's, crossing the 't's and filling in the gaps in the picture you are building up of the patient's problem (see Figure 4.10).

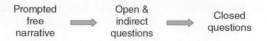

FIGURE 4.10

Here are some examples:

- 'You mentioned you had some pain' *(narrative prompt)*
- 'What was the pain like?' *(open question)*
- 'It would help me to know how the pain came on' *(indirect question)*
- 'When did the pain start? Did it spread to your neck or arms?' *(closed questions)*

As you move from prompts to open questions to closed questions, the information you glean becomes more specific, but you risk losing unexpected, possibly significant, additional details.

This sequencing strategy is only a suggestion, a 'broad brush' generalisation. How you order your questions and in what form you ask them will depend partly on the particulars of the case, partly on the personality of the individual patient and partly on your own consulting style. However, one legacy of the way you were taught to take a history at medical school will almost certainly be an over-reliance on closed questions. So here is a suggestion as to how you can train yourself to be more comfortable with the more open-ended approach appropriate in general practice.

Watch a video recording of some of your consultations. Make a note of how many times you ask a closed question, compared with the number of open or indirect ones. This will raise your awareness of how 'closed question-dependent' you are. Then see if you can think of an indirect or open question alternative you could have asked instead. (If you are terribly camera-shy, you could even do this while watching someone else's consultations.)

Physical examination

The body tells its story even more reliably than the tongue – provided you ask it the right questions and know what to do with the answers.

If – heaven forbid! – you were a hospital-oriented doctor looking for a stick to beat general practice with, you might seize upon the average GP's competence at conducting a physical examination. Good practice, you might piously insist, requires that every organ system of every patient should be examined thoroughly and systematically, so that no abnormality can escape detection. The way GPs typically examine their patients, you might assert, falls well short of this ideal. And (I'm pleased to say) you would be right. If you were a GP defending yourself against this charge, you might point out the utter impracticality of spending 30 minutes or so routinely examining every patient from top to toe; the way many conditions present before there are any reliable physical signs; the consequences for your time and reputation of asking every patient to take their clothes off ... I hope you would also argue that physical disease as evidenced by physical abnormalities is only a part of the more comprehensive picture of the problem each patient presents for your attention.

Nevertheless, the importance of detecting relevant physical signs where they exist cannot be overestimated. People suffer, or even die, if you don't. So, both in real-life general practice and in the SCA, a three-way compromise has to be struck between thoroughness, relevance and significance.

My personal opinion is that, whenever you perform any kind of physical examination in general practice, you should be ready to answer two questions that the patient might reasonably ask: *Why are you doing this?* and *What are you looking for?* Indeed, it's not a bad idea to tell the patient this information even if they don't ask for it. Usually, you will be looking for the presence or absence of clinical features that would support or refute diagnostic possibilities that have occurred to you in the conversational part of the consultation. But sometimes we examine patients in a more exploratory kind of way, in case we come across some pointer to a diagnosis we hadn't thought of, as when, for example, unexpectedly noticing a goitre reminds us that thyroid disease can cause menorrhagia. Sometimes, too, we examine a patient chiefly because they want or expect it, for reassurance or to confirm that we are taking their symptoms seriously.

You are a GP; no one expects you to be able to examine every organ system with the rigour, fluency and expertise of a consultant in the relevant specialty. But it *is* reasonable to expect you to know how to test for and recognise signs of conditions that are common and/or serious. It is easy to let one's skills in physical examination atrophy through disuse; the deterioration all the more likely since abnormal findings are less frequently encountered in general practice than in hospital.

The timing of any physical examination – whether you perform it during the course of the Doctor's part or at its conclusion – largely depends on the nature of the problem. If a patient comes in, shows you a ganglion on the wrist, and asks, 'What's this?'—it would be silly not to examine it there and then. If on the other hand a patient tells you anxiously about her postmenopausal bleeding, weight loss and family history of cancer, it would be insensitive not to allow the full expression of her story and the full clarification of her symptoms before proceeding to examine her.

Be cautious about multitasking – examining the patient while at the same time carrying on verbal data-gathering. Very occasionally, the trust implied by the patient's allowing you to touch them will lead to further revelation of important information. But this is rare; your attention is, or should be, on conducting the examination, and the patient is more likely to be wondering whether it's going to hurt or tickle.

Physical examination in the SCA

An important change in the SCA, compared with its predecessors, the CSA and RCA, is that your ability to conduct a physical examination is no longer tested in this component of the MRCGP. This follows acceptance by the General Medical Council, which oversees all medical licensing exams, that it is not possible reliably to assess a doctor's competence in physical examination by means of a small number of remote consultations where the 'patient' is a role-player. Instead, this vital medical skill is now tested in the Workplace-Based Assessment.

Nevertheless, it is entirely possible in an SCA case being conducted over a phone or video link that you might want to gather some data about physical findings. Sometimes you can do this simply by asking questions, such as, 'Does your swollen knee feel hot to the touch?' or 'Can you put your hand behind your head without pain?' or 'If you smile, does your face look lopsided?' Most people have a thermometer in their home and could tell you their temperature if asked. And some patients with chronic diseases may have the kit necessary to report their blood pressure or blood glucose level. In such cases, the role-player will have been briefed to provide you with the information you ask for.

If you feel that an actual hands-on physical examination is necessary and you plan to call the patient in for a face-to-face consultation, it is reasonable for the examiner to expect you to tell your patient why you need to do this and to explain briefly what the examination will consist of. You might say, for example, 'I'd like you to bring a sample of urine in to the surgery so that I can test it for any signs of infection. And I'll also need to examine your prostate gland, which will involve my gently slipping a finger into your back passage to see if your prostate feels normal.'

Adding your own agenda to the consultation

In addition to whatever problem has prompted the patient to attend, it is increasingly common for the doctor to bring agenda to the consultation. Although it has long been common practice to slip into a consultation a casual 'When did you last have a tetanus booster?' or 'While you've got your shirt off, I'll just check your blood pressure,' doctor-initiated agenda has reached a new order of magnitude and acquired a more pressing priority since the advent of the QOF in 2004.[4] In many real-life consultations now, the computer will be nagging you for information or action with the irritating persistence of a four-year-old in a sweet shop, including a panoply of clinical parameters relating to chronic disease management, cervical smears, vaccinations, body mass index, smoking status and so on. Or you might find yourself being told to undertake a formal depression screen, detect problem drinking or document smoking cessation advice.[5] Although a case can be made that some of this is in the overall interests of the patient's health,[6] it can be difficult or disruptive to make time for it in an already crowded consultation that is ostensibly devoted to the patient's agenda.

There are probably two points in the consultation where, if you wish, you can create an opportunity to introduce your own agenda with minimum disruption. The first is during the Doctor's part, where you have control of the questioning, and the other is at the end of the Shared part, where, once the patient's agenda has been addressed, you could change the subject and have what is, in effect, a second 'mini-consultation' on the topic of your choosing.

As to how to do it, you already know how to steer the consultation if you want to: you turn in a receipt. You say to the patient, in effect, 'Thank you for that, but now I'd like to talk about something else.' The more seamless you can make the transition, the better. So in the Doctor's part, you might say, 'You told me you don't smoke; how much do you drink?' or 'It's good that you

---

[4] The Quality and Outcomes Framework (QOF) was part of a package of changes introduced to the NHS General Medical Services contract with effect from April 2004. According to official Department of Health literature, 'the QOF is a system to remunerate general practices for providing good quality care to their patients …(It) measures achievement against a range of evidence-based indicators, with points and payments awarded according to the level of achievement.' Indicators cover four domains: clinical, public health, patient experience, and records and system. The Department insists that QOF 'is not about performance management of general practices but about resourcing and rewarding good practice … (It) is only one measure of the quality of clinical care provided to patients … A lower quality achievement does not necessarily mean that patients are receiving poorer quality care.' Nevertheless, since more points mean more income, the QOF for the first time introduced a financial incentive for GPs not to make the patient's agenda their sole priority.

[5] The range and details of QOF-driven information and other doctor-led agenda vary from time to time. The examples given here are not necessarily comprehensive or up to date.

[6] It isn't all in the patient's interests, however. NHS administrative bodies such as Clinical Commissioning Groups increasingly seek to impose their own agenda on the consultation, encouraging the GP, for example, to conform to local prescribing or referral policies, or to document information which is clinically irrelevant but financially lucrative. For instance, at the time of writing, entering a diagnosis of 'sprain' can result in a computer prompt to complete a 'minor injury' template to allow the practice to claim an additional payment, even though the 'sprain' may actually have been the patient's pretext to discuss depression. Perhaps more worryingly, in view of doubts over the security of electronic records, in October 2017, NHS England proposed that GPs should ask about, and record, patients' sexual orientation 'at every face to face contact with the patient, where no record of this data already exists.' Many patients would give a four-word response to such an enquiry – 'Mind your own business.' Others might insert an additional word before 'business.'

try and look after your health; but incidentally, I see you're overdue to have a smear test.' If your own doctor-led agenda involves a substantial change of topic, it is probably best to leave it until the end of the Shared part. An example: 'So we'll get these blood tests done and I'll see you in two weeks. Now, while you're here, I see we're due to check on how your asthma is doing.'

A question of style and values

Imagine this: just as you are coming towards the end of a perfectly satisfactory consultation, the patient unexpectedly says, 'While I'm here, Doctor, could I ask you about something else?' Don't you feel a bit irritated because the unwritten rules of the consultation are being broken? A bit abused, because the patient is taking advantage of what has been a good doctor–patient relationship? You don't want to say *Yes*, but you don't like to say *No*. Probably you think *What a shame, just as we were getting on so well.* You ask yourself, *Is this going to be the main reason they came?* If it's something quick, you'll probably deal with it, but rather grudgingly or with bad grace. If it's something more complicated, you'll probably ask the patient to make another appointment, which they will do, but with rather bad grace.

Now reverse the situation: imagine yourself to be a patient, and a perfectly satisfactory consultation with your doctor appears to be drawing to a close. Then, unexpectedly, the doctor says, 'While you're here, could I ask you about something else?' How would you react? There's no reason why patients should welcome a doctor's unexpected agenda any more than the doctor would welcome theirs.

There is no 'right' answer to the question of whether or not you, the doctor, should introduce your own agenda into an otherwise patient-led consultation. Both options have consequences. If you *don't*, some potentially valuable health promotion opportunities may be lost, some routine clinical information may go unrecorded, some performance targets possibly get missed, and your relations with the practice management team become temporarily strained. If you *do*, you risk alienating your patient by giving the impression that you are prioritising your own interests over theirs. There is also a danger that trying to work your own hidden agenda into the consultation may lead you to do less than full justice to that of the patient.

Several factors may affect your decision: how much time you've got; how clinically important your agenda is; whether the patient is in a suitable frame of mind to accept a change of topic[7]; and whether you can make the

---

[7] I recall once, in an old-style MRCGP oral exam, asking a candidate how he would deal with a patient who had collapsed in the waiting room, and being told that his immediate management would include checking when her next smear test was due. And, from the look on his face, he expected to be given credit for this response.

transition reasonably seamless. But ultimately it's a question of style and values – of knowing what kind of doctor you want to be and your own view of what a GP's priorities should be. It's decisions like this that test your commitment to what I believe ought to be an over-riding principle: that you are there for the patient's benefit, not they for yours.

Knowing when to stop

At medical school, we learned lists of questions to ask as part of taking a comprehensive history, and the habit of lengthy doctor-led questioning dies hard. We always seem able to think of one more question, and it's hard to resist the temptation to ask it. But in general practice, in the interests of time and efficiency, we have to learn to discriminate between what information is essential to obtain, what is relevant but not vital and what is superfluous, so that we don't waste time pursuing unnecessary details just for the sake of completeness.

In any consultation, but particularly in the SCA, it's important to be able to draw a line under your data-gathering in order to move on to the 'what-are-we-going-to-do-about-it?' Shared part. I've made the point elsewhere in this book, but it bears repeating: most SCA cases will entail at least 5 minutes-worth of management, and not leaving time for it will lose you a third of the available marks. In real life, where the clock is not ticking quite so relentlessly, you can afford to stretch the Doctor's part if you wish. But in a fixed-length SCA case, you should, as a rough guide, be moving on to decision-making and management no later than 6 or 7 minutes into the consultation.

Probably the main thing that makes us prolong the Doctor's part is the fear of missing something important. This fear is particularly strong when, as in an exam, our performance is under scrutiny. It is perfectly understandable that an SCA candidate will worry that they have completely missed the point of the case, and will therefore keep asking questions in the hope of uncovering the 'real' problem.

Two strategies can be useful to reassure you that it is OK to move on from data-gathering to management planning. The first is to summarise – offer the patient a succinct version of what you understand to be the reason for the consultation, the details you have elicited about the problem, and your findings on examination, if any. If the patient accepts your summary, as when the patient in the above exchange says 'Exactly,' you can take this at face value. In the SCA, the role-player will not lie or try to mislead you.

Another strategy, which can be very reassuring in the SCA if you have any nagging doubts, is to say to the patient something like, 'We ought to move on now, but before we do, is there anything else you think I need to know in order to help you?' Or even, 'I want to be sure I haven't missed anything important about your problem, so please tell me if you think I have.'

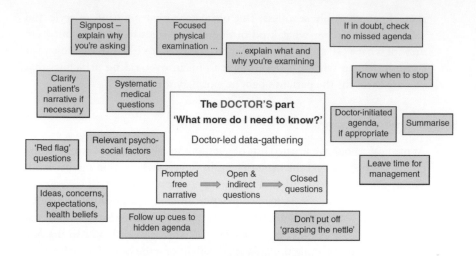

FIGURE 4.11

One additional reason for lingering in the Doctor's part, sometimes seen in SCA candidates, might be described as 'reluctance to grasp the nettle.' If it becomes clear in the early part of the consultation that managing the case is going to be difficult, it is tempting to put off the hard part – to delay grasping the nettle – in the vain hope that somehow the difficulty will vanish or the examiner won't notice that you didn't get round to tackling it. It won't, and they will. This situation often arises if the case exposes a knowledge gap, e.g. how to explain the inheritance of cystic fibrosis, or requires a contentious ethical decision, e.g. whether to breach a young person's confidentiality. I think the best tactic in such circumstances is to explain your difficulty or dilemma out loud,[8] and say, for example, 'I'm a bit hazy about this, so I'd like to do some homework and then see you again when I can be sure of the facts,' or 'This is a difficult situation, and I'd like to get the advice of one of my colleagues.' Although these responses are not as meritorious as if you had been able to deal with the matter there and then, they at least allow you to move on and make a workable plan for completing the case. If the examiner sees that you don't know what to do, the unspoken question to be answered, and for which marks can be given, is 'Do you know what to do when you don't know what to do?'

Figure 4.11 summarises the key points that will help you make a success of the Doctor's part.

---

[8] 'Thinking aloud' can be an extremely useful strategy throughout the consultation. We'll return to it in detail when we consider how to make a success of the Shared part.

EXAM POINT: Data-gathering and diagnosis

Don't assume, just because you see the word '*diagnosis*' in the heading of one of the SCA marking domains, that there will be a formal biomedical diagnosis in every case and that you will be expected to make it. Very often, in general practice, there *isn't* one. 'Tired all the time', or 'Worried about cancer', or 'Possible domestic violence??' are not, strictly speaking, diagnoses. What there *is,* however, in every case is a *problem*, and your challenge is to identify it in sufficient physical, psychological, emotional and social detail for you to be able to reach a plan for dealing with it.

Possibly 'assessment' or 'evaluation' or 'problem identification' would be better words than *diagnosis* to describe what the examiners are looking for. If there *is* a physical diagnosis or differential diagnosis in a particular case, it is, of course, important that you should make it. But, since this is an exam in general practice, your assessment will also include insights into the patient's situation and context, their thoughts and feelings and the impact of the problem on their life.

Transitioning from the Doctor's part to the Shared part

We come now to the consultation's second transition point, where the focus switches from 'working out what the problem is' to 'working out what is to be done about it' (Figure 4.12). You've got as much information as you need to make your diagnosis or assessment (or as much as you're probably going to get), and it's time to move on to decision-making and action-planning.

Compared to the previous transition, when the Patient's part morphed into the Doctor's part, the transition from the Doctor's part to the Shared part is a more substantial and significant change of gear. Until now, you and the

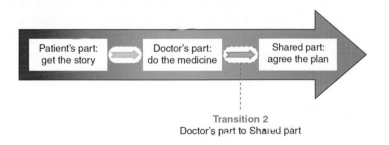

Transition 2
Doctor's part to Shared part

FIGURE 4.12

patient have taken it in turns to be active and passive. In the Patient's part, you encouraged the patient to take the lead in giving information; yours was a more passive, non-directive facilitatory role. Then, in the Doctor's part, the roles were reversed, with you leading and the patient responding. But in the Shared part, both of you have to move beyond ideas of leading and following and establish a more collaborative 'relationship of equals.'

This is not easy for either of you. We doctors are very accustomed to telling people what we think is in their best interests. We are in the habit of giving advice, and by and large, we expect it to be taken. And why should it *not* be? After all, underlying our professional opinions is a weight of medical experience, expertise and evidence that vastly exceeds the information available to the average patient, Doctor Google notwithstanding. But, for a variety of social, historical and cultural reasons, the traditional expectation that 'doctor's orders' are to be followed unquestioningly is no longer acceptable, and rightly so. Modern medical practice, especially general practice, and particularly the action-planning stage of the consultation, requires of us doctors a 'suspension of authority' that doesn't always come easily.

For the Shared part to be genuinely collaborative, suspension of the doctor's authority has to be matched by what we might call a 'suspension of deference' by the patient. The patient needs to be willing to participate and contribute on equal terms and accept some responsibility for the outcome, and this doesn't always come easily either. After all, to be a patient is almost by definition to be in need of guidance. And during the Doctor's part, the patient has effectively been rehearsed in adopting a subservient position. So as the consultation enters its final phase, doctor and patient both have to make an abrupt change in mindset. Frustration awaits if one of you is left stranded in data-generating mode while the other has moved on in their mind to action-planning. And it isn't only the patient who can always think of 'just one more thing' to mention. Some SCA candidates, whether through fear of missing the point or uncertainty about their management options, can be particularly reluctant to draw a line under the Doctor's part. To them, I would say, 'Be confident. When you think you understand the problem, move on. Don't keep going back to ask just one more question. If you *have* missed something important, the patient will let you know.'

Making the transition

To ensure you're both in sync, I think it's helpful to signpost clearly and explicitly when you're ready for the consultation to move into its 'What-shall-we-do-about-the-problem?' phase. And you know how to do this:

you 'steer' by turning a receipt. You acknowledge what has gone before and then indicate what is to happen next. In effect, you say to the patient, 'I think I understand what the problem is. Now let's discuss what we should do about it.'

Naturally, you won't use these exact words every time. You'll tailor what you say to the specifics of the case. Sometimes – if the case is very straightforward or if it's obvious that no further details of the problem are necessary – the receipt can be brief, even non-existent. In appropriate circumstances, all that might need saying could be, 'I can see you're not ready to go back to work yet. You'll be needing another certificate,' or even 'Okay, let's talk about treatment now.'

With more complex problems, a summary is an effective receipt to signal the end of data-gathering. Even if you summarised after the Patient's part, and especially if you have carried out a physical examination in the Doctor's part, it is worth briefly updating your summary to make sure that you both start the Shared part on the same footing. On the other hand, don't summarise just for the sake of it. There is a danger of summarising becoming as much of an irritating cliché as 'doing the ICE'; only do it if it feels helpful as a way of gathering your thoughts before moving on.

Remember David Wren, the man with indigestion? To him, for example, you might say: 'So, Mr Wren; you've told me about the symptoms you've been getting for the last few months, which you thought were just indigestion, until your wife showed you that article about stomach cancer, which understandably has got you both worried. I'm pleased to say there's nothing in what you've told me that worries me. And I've not found anything wrong when I examined you ...' Then Mr Wren will nod or say, 'That's right.' And now both you and he are ready to discuss the next steps in his management. We'll explore how to do this shortly. But first, we need to make sure that you too are in the right frame of mind for the Shared part of the consultation to be a *genuinely* shared piece of decision-making.

'Plan A'

You've heard the story, you've asked your questions, you've examined if necessary, you've made your assessment, you reckon you probably know what the problem is. So, of course, before anything more is said, you've already started to work out a possible plan of action. You've begun to think ahead to how, if it was left up to you, you would like to manage the situation. What we might call 'Plan A' is forming in your mind.

In Mr Wren's case, for instance, you might be thinking: *Almost certainly not cancer; maybe just lifestyle, or reflux, or a peptic ulcer. I'll need to check for H. pylori – is that a blood test or a breath test? But there's a lot of anxiety about cancer.*

So I'll get him to bring his wife when he comes back for the test results. He could try a PPI in the meantime …

It's very comforting to have a Plan A at this stage of the consultation. It's like feeling the sand under your feet when swimming in the sea and realising that you're not out of your depth. It means that at least you're not going to suffer the indignity of having no idea what to do next. But beware. Earlier in this book, I cautioned against 'premature medicalisation' – fixating too soon on a medical interpretation of the patient's problem before you had sufficient information. Premature commitment to your Plan A can be equally dangerous. Plan A might not ultimately prove to be as good as you first think it is. Like teenage puppy love, it's possible to be so infatuated with Plan A that it dominates your every thought and blinds you to other, perhaps more fruitful, possibilities.

Your Plan A may well be perfectly sensible. After all, it will have emerged from a combination of your own clinical knowledge and experience with whatever insight you have gained into the patient's particular circumstances. But it is still only a possibility, capable of being modified, improved, abandoned or replaced.

Your Plan A for Mr Wren – test for *H. pylori* and start him on omeprazole – is indeed perfectly sensible. But it might not be what Mr Wren has in mind. *His* Plan A might be for you to refer him for an endoscopy, because that's what it said in the magazine article about stomach cancer that got his wife so worried. He hadn't liked to mention this earlier in the consultation because he knows doctors dislike their patients telling them what to do, and besides, in the back of his mind is a fear, which he knows is irrational, that testing for cancer somehow makes having it more likely.

So as you embark on the Shared part of the consultation, keep your Plan A, if you have one, under wraps for the time being. Don't produce it with a flourish like a rabbit out of a magician's hat. At this stage, Plan A is an option, not a manifesto.

Making a success of the Shared part

[A]

It seems to me that we have reached a gathering point, and I want to take stock and tell you where I, personally, have got to. In my imagination, I've brought you on a journey through the consultation. We started on the patient's home ground, then moved on into our own more familiar medical territory, building up as we went along an appreciation of why it is that we are travelling at all. And I've told you where we're going next. Our destination, all being well, is an outcome where everyone involved is as satisfied as possible under the circumstances. I feel a bit like a guide, showing a party

The SHARED part

'What management plan will we both be happy with?'

- Explaining
- Discussing
- Respecting patient's preferences and health beliefs
- Considering options
- Collaborative decision-making
- Action planning
- Checking for understanding
- Safety-netting and follow-up plans

FIGURE 4.13

of tourists round the sights of my favourite city, holding up my umbrella to signify *Follow me*, and stopping from time to time to point out landmarks and features of interest. Figure 4.13 shows some of the commonly recommended points on the itinerary of the Shared part.

That's where *I* am, but I don't know where *you* are. I hope you're still with me. But it's possible you might already be running ahead of me, or you might have got bored and gone off in some other direction of your own. If that *is* the case, this being a book and not a real-life conversation, I have no way of knowing. And you can't let me know, for the same reason. If we were face to face, I could ask you to tell me your own thoughts about how to finesse the 'what-shall-we-do-about-it?' Shared part of the consultation. You could tell me where you think the difficulties lie or what tips or strategies you have found useful in the past. And I could tell you how, in my opinion, the Shared part is the most difficult one to bring off. I could explain why I think some of the standard advice is not as helpful as it might be, and I could suggest what I think are some better ways of bringing the consultation to a satisfactory conclusion. You would probably have some questions you would like me to answer, which I might or might not have anticipated, and, face to face, I could do my best to address them. Face to face, we could have a conversation where we could be sure of talking about exactly the things that mattered to you personally.

[B]

But without that two-way exchange of information, all I can do – my 'Plan A,' if you like – is continue to set out my thoughts and suggestions in the best way I can, hoping that you'll find them useful. And all you can do is read (and hopefully understand) what I'm saying, but with no guarantee that it will actually fit your own individual interests.

You'll perhaps have noticed that I marked off the first two paragraphs of this section from [A] to [B]. Read them again and see if you can notice what I'm doing. That passage is as close as I can come to 'thinking aloud' on the page: telling you how I see things at this point in the book and suggesting how helpful it would have been if you had been able to respond in person, telling me your own thoughts in return.

The shortcomings of the virtual conversation you and I are having through print have a lesson for the real conversation *you* have face to face with your patient. It's better if you can tell each other what you're thinking. In the consulting room, for you as the doctor to speak your thoughts out loud so that the patient can know what's in your mind as you begin the Shared part, is going to be my top tip for making a success of the decision-making phase of the consultation. But all in good time. Perhaps we should start by asking an obvious question.

Does shared decision-making matter?

The cynical answer is that patients who don't feel involved in decisions that affect them are more likely to become disgruntled, be uncooperative, and make complaints. If you're an SCA candidate, an equally cynical answer is that a third of each station's marks are for management, and another third are for how you relate to the patient and conduct the consultation; and shared decision-making spans both domains.

But it's not just the defence organisations and the RCGP who want to see patients actively participating in decisions about their own management. Other official bodies are keen on it too. The General Medical Council, for instance, sets out in paralysing detail everything you are supposed to discuss with your patient before any course of action is agreed (see Figure 4.14).

As I write, the National Institute for Health and Care Excellence (NICE) is developing its own guidelines on this topic. A background document states that

> Shared decision making is a collaborative process through which a healthcare professional supports a person to reach a decision about their care … It involves healthcare professionals working together with people who use services and their families and carers to choose tests, treatments, management or support packages based on evidence and personal informed preferences, health beliefs, and values. This involves making sure the person has a good understanding of the risks, benefits and possible consequences of different options through discussion and information sharing. This joint process empowers people to make decisions about the treatment and care that is right for them at that time (including doing nothing).

GMC guidance* on 'Sharing information and discussing treatment options'

7 The exchange of information between doctor and patient is central to good decision-making. How much information you share with patients will vary, depending on their individual circumstances. You should tailor your approach to discussions with patients according to:
   a. their needs, wishes and priorities
   b. their level of knowledge about, and understanding of, their condition, prognosis and the treatment options
   c. the nature of their condition
   d. the complexity of the treatment, and
   e. the nature and level of risk associated with the investigation or treatment.
8 You should not make assumptions about:
   a. the information a patient might want or need
   b. the clinical or other factors a patient might consider significant, or
   c. a patient's level of knowledge or understanding of what is proposed.
9 You must give patients the information they want or need about:
   a. the diagnosis and prognosis
   b any uncertainties about the diagnosis or prognosis, including options for further investigations
   c. options for treating or managing the condition, including the option not to treat
   d. the purpose of any proposed investigation or treatment and what it will involve
   e. the potential benefits, risks and burdens, and the likelihood of success, for each option; this should include information, if available, about whether the benefits or risks are affected by which organisation or doctor is chosen to provide care
   f. whether a proposed investigation or treatment is part of a research programme or is an innovative treatment designed specifically for their benefit[4]
   g. the people who will be mainly responsible for and involved in their care, what their roles are, and to what extent students may be involved
   h. their right to refuse to take part in teaching or research
   i. their right to seek a second opinion
   j. any bills they will have to pay
   k. any conflicts of interest that you, or your organisation, may have
   l. any treatments that you believe have greater potential benefit for the patient than those you or your organisation can offer.
10 You should explore these matters with patients, listen to their concerns, ask for the respect their views, and encourage them to ask questions.
11 You should check whether patients have understood the information they have been given, and whether or not they would like more information before making a decision. You must make it clear that they can change their mind about a decision.

*From *Consent: patients and doctors making decisions together*

FIGURE 4.14

The advocates of shared decision-making are long on rhetoric but relatively short on evidence that it benefits clinical outcomes. Nevertheless, there are some indications that a sense of partnership between patient and doctor improves compliance, speeds recovery from illness, reduces referral rates, increases patient satisfaction and reduces doctors' work-related stress.[9]

Within the medical profession, however, opinion remains divided. Responding to an essay on shared decision-making in the *British Medical Journal*,[10] one correspondent wrote,

> The complexity of shared decision-making is under-rated. Doing it as an ethical duty is not inspiring, particularly when patients don't seem to get the point or want to throw the ball back to the doctor. Shared decision-making should be part of the healing process — a remedy to restore the patient's autonomous capacity, which is reduced when ill.' Someone else, on the other hand, saw it differently: 'The basic problem with shared decision-making is that it has always been a matter of ideology rather than evidence … Asymmetry is at the heart of doctor–patient interactions. Doctors have expertise that patients want or need but do not have for themselves. When doctors decline to act as experts, patients are reduced to interactional strategies that try to divine clues from gnomic utterances.

My own view, for what it's worth, is that making a plan to deal with a patient's problem should be a shared enterprise simply because it's 'right'; it's the right way for two people to relate to each other in order for both of them to be satisfied with the outcome. The inevitable asymmetry of medical knowledge and experience confers on us, I think, a duty to balance our expertise with humility and respect. This means not 'doing shared decision-making' in a routine, formulaic way, just because some pundit says we should. It means recognising that different patients need to be involved in different ways and to different extents. Paying lip service to shared decision-making isn't good enough; if you're going to do it at all, it needs to be genuine. And that can be difficult.

Why is the Shared part difficult?

Most of us receive our basic medical training within a hospital-orientated, doctor-centred tradition. We learn the 'medical model' of how we should

---

[9] See, for example, Fong J. and Longnecker N. (2010). Doctor–patient communication: a review. Ochsner J. 10:38–43.

[10] Maskrey N. (2019). Shared decision-making: why is progress so slow? BMJ. 367:l6762.

think and act as doctors. It's a familiar catechism, hard-wired into us: history, examination, investigations, diagnosis and treatment. The unspoken assumption is that the doctor is in charge of the process from start to finish; the doctor is responsible for making the right diagnosis and prescribing the right management. The patient's role is purely passive one; essentially, it's to follow the doctor's orders. Of course, the reality is not quite so Stalinist. Most doctors don't behave as arrogantly or as autocratically as this, and most patients wouldn't stand for it if they tried. Nonetheless, a doctor-centred way of consulting is deeply engrained in us, and we tend to revert to it under pressure, such as when we're puzzled, or stressed, or uncertain, or doing an exam.

But times have changed. The days of the doctor as benevolent dictator or fount of all wisdom have thankfully all but gone. No profession is beyond accountability, and nor should it be. As consumers of medical services, patients are no longer willing to accept unquestioned, with forelock-tugging gratitude, whatever decisions a doctor chooses to hand down, no matter how well-intentioned. Moreover, patients now have not only the confidence to expect a more egalitarian relationship with their doctors but also, thanks to the internet and digital technology, access to the information necessary to back it up.

It is not always easy for doctors to accommodate their consulting style to this shift in cultural norms. Patient-centredness does not always come naturally, especially to someone trained in a country or healthcare system where a more deferential or reverential attitude towards the medical profession prevails. Some doctors, too, for reasons of their own psychology, feel threatened by patients who wish to participate as equals in the consultation. There will always be some colleagues for whom, although they say otherwise, patient-centredness is something of an act, a veneer that, under pressure, will wear thin and reveal an underlying preference for an authoritarian way of consulting.

Much more common, however, is the doctor who, in all honesty, wants to practise in a patient-centred way, valuing the patient's contribution and respecting their right to exercise informed choice, and yet who finds it hard to put these good intentions into practice in real time with real patients. Here, more than at any other time in the consultation, a gap can open up between rhetoric and reality, between aspiration and performance.

There is no shortage of guidance about how to make a success of the action-planning part of the consultation. This is summarised in Figure 4.15, which shows a doctor whose head is buzzing as he reminds himself of everything he means to do in order to give the patient a genuine say in the decision-making. *Don't be doctor-centred*, he tells himself.

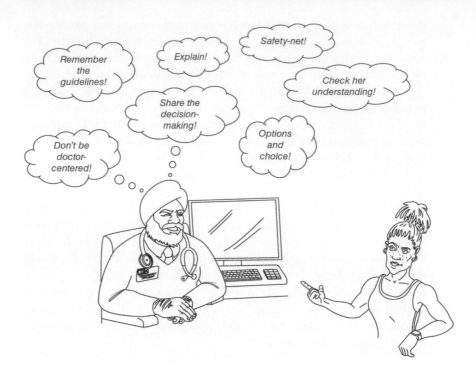

FIGURE 4.15

But try to keep the clinical guidelines. Take time to explain the situation to the patient, in language she will understand. Tell her about the various alternative options available to her. Allow her to choose, and respect her choice. The more involved she feels, the more likely she is to agree and cooperate with whatever is decided. And when you've got a plan, make sure she understands it. Give her the chance to ask questions. Oh, and don't forget about follow-up and safety-netting ….

All this excellent advice really boils down to nothing more than *Treat the patient as you would like to be treated yourself.* But in the professional setting of the consulting room, it is hard to do this with the same spontaneity as you would if you were talking to a friend or family member in more relaxed surroundings. The strain of 'trying to be natural on purpose' can easily make one's attempts at patient–centredness sound forced or insincere. What's more, it is understandable if, at this point in the consultation, a bit of latent resentment at having to be patient-centred occasionally creeps in. After all, you are a trained medical professional, and you *do* have some expertise – almost certainly more expertise in matters of health than does your patient. And you probably already have a 'Plan A' in your mind based on sound medical knowledge and experience. Surely your advice ought to carry more weight than the less well-informed views of a patient who, after all, has come to see you in order to benefit from your opinion? And let's be honest, patients' preferences and expectations are not always sensible or realistic, are they?

In the literature, there is a broad consensus about how to conduct the decision-making and action-planning phases of the consultation successfully. We'll look at some of the standard recommendations now and see how best to put them into practice. But we'll find that it's not as easy as it sounds. Much of the advice that seems fine in principle has to be somewhat qualified and compromised in real life. After that (spoiler alert!), I'll describe a strategy – thinking aloud – that I believe offers the best chance of bringing the consultation to a genuinely patient-centred conclusion.

Let's start with something you have to do on practically every occasion.

Explaining

Two questions arise immediately: *What do you need to explain*, and *how are you to do it*? As to *what* needs explaining, there are things the patient wants to know, and there are things you want to tell them. These are not necessarily the same.

As you reach the point in the consultation where the agenda switches from *What's the problem?* to *What shall we do about it?*—try to imagine the questions that will be in the patient's mind.

In 1981, a medical anthropologist called Cecil Helman published what has become known as the 'folk model' of illness.[11] Helman suggested that a patient bringing a problem to a doctor is seeking the answers to six questions (Figure 4.16):

1   *What has happened?* What has caused the problem? What has gone wrong? Is there a name for what I've got?

2   *Why has it happened?* Is there a reason, or is it just one of those things? Is it because of something I've done? Or *not* done? Could it be stress? Or just in my mind?

3   *Why to me?* Is it my age? My way of life? My job? In my genes?

4   *Why now?* Why hasn't it happened before? Has it been brought on by something else going on in my life at the moment?

---

[11] Helman CG. (1981). Diseases versus illness in general practice. J R Coll Gen Pract. 13:548–552.

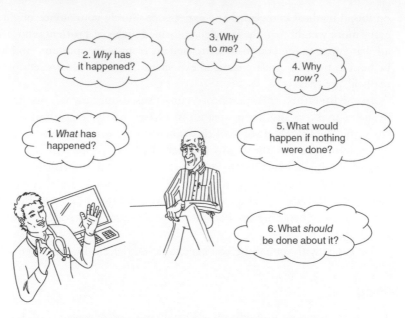

Six questions the patient wants answers to (*after Helman*)

FIGURE 4.16

5   *What would happen if nothing were done?* Is it serious? Could I die? Or will it just get better on its own? How long would it last? What could be the long-term effects? How is it going to affect my family?

6   *What should be done about it?* Have I done the right thing by coming to see you? Are you the right person to help me? Do I need any investigations? How can it be treated? What are my options? What do you advise?

Obviously, the particulars of each individual case will determine what your patient's chief concerns are. But if you have been paying proper attention during the Patient's and Doctor's parts, it shouldn't be too hard to know what to emphasise in your explanation.

To make this discussion more concrete, let's see how it might apply to David Wren, the 40-year-old man with dyspepsia. Mr Wren, if you remember, has been generally healthy until a few months ago, when he began to suffer from what he calls 'indigestion,' relieved by over-the-counter antacids. He has consulted you because his wife showed him a magazine article about stomach cancer, and now he's worried he might have been ignoring potentially serious symptoms. Let's assume he is otherwise well, with no 'red flag' symptoms. Let's also assume you have examined him and found no abnormal signs in his abdomen. So here he sits in your consulting room, anxiously waiting to see what you are going to say. You can readily imagine the thoughts racing through his brain:

> *Please don't let it be cancer. I'm glad I got it off my chest, though. The doctor doesn't seem particularly worried. Perhaps I am just wasting her time. If it is cancer, I don't know how I'll cope. Or Angela. Maybe she should have come with me. It's probably just stress from work. It's a wake-up call; this time I really will stop smoking. I hope I don't have to go to hospital. I don't like the sound of that tube thing they put down you, like it said in the article...*

Meanwhile, you the doctor also have your own list of things you want to explain to your patient. These might include:

- your assessment of what the problem is;
- your diagnosis or differential diagnosis;
- your response to the patient's own ideas or expectations;
- your preferred 'Plan A' for what to do next;
- other realistic management or treatment options;
- any constraints on your management, such as prescribing policies or referral guidelines;
- any information the patient is likely to need in order to make an informed choice about management options.

In Mr Wren's case, for example, you might want to tell him that:

- There's nothing about his symptoms or examination that makes you think he has stomach cancer;
- in fact, you're 99% sure he doesn't.
- It's much more likely he has a stomach infection called *H. pylori*, which is common, easy to diagnose with a blood test, and easy to treat.
- Alternatively, he could have reflux of stomach acid into his oesophagus.
- The only way to be really sure he doesn't have cancer would be to refer him for an endoscopy,
- but you don't think it's necessary.
- What you'd rather do is a test for *H. pylori*, see him together with his wife when you have the results, and try an antacid medication in the meantime.
- You can give him a leaflet with some information about dyspepsia, which he could show his wife;
- but he must let you know if ever he gets any 'red flag' symptoms.

Somehow, you have to put together an explanation that covers the patient's questions, spoken and unspoken, and your own medical agenda as well. This is a tall order. But it is important to do it as well as you possibly can. The data-gathering part of the consultation was concerned with getting the patient's 'story so far.' Now, your explanation and the discussion that follows it are, in effect, writing the next chapter in that story. What you say will not be remembered in word-for-word detail; the patient will translate what he can recall of it into his own words, which he will subsequently go over in his own mind and pass on to family and friends. Here are some suggestions for how you can give your explanation the best chance of being understood and remembered.

- Use words and language your patient is likely to understand. Avoid jargon, bearing in mind that some of the medical words we use without a second thought, such as *hormone* or *inflammation*, may be unfamiliar to a lay person. But try not to sound patronising either.

- Make your most important points (or the ones that are most important to the patient) first, e.g. 'The first thing to say, Mr Wren, is that I don't think you have cancer.'

- 'Signpost' and emphasise your key points, as if you were giving your explanation paragraph headings, e.g. 'Now let me tell you what I think is causing your symptoms.'

- Break down your explanation into separate manageable 'chunks' of information, pausing in between to let what you have said sink in.

- Notice how the patient is reacting to what you are saying, so that you can tell whether it is being understood. Give the patient opportunities to ask for clarification or put a question.

- If necessary, check for understanding by asking, 'Is that clear? Is this making sense to you? Would you like me to write this down for you?'

- Link what you are saying to what you have already learned about the patient's ideas, concerns and expectations, e.g. 'If it was the only way to put your mind at rest, I could always get you to see a specialist. But actually, I think you're right – this isn't anything very serious.'

- Resist the temptation to 'do a knowledge dump' and deliver a lecture on, for example, 'Everything I know about proton pump inhibitors.' Remember, you are talking to a worried human being, not reading out an undergraduate essay. Keep it relevant.

- If it helps – and *only* if it helps – reinforce what you are saying with a leaflet or a quick hand-drawn sketch or diagram. But beware of digging a hole for yourself by attempting a graphic of the anatomy of the carpal tunnel or the inheritance of cystic fibrosis.

Remember, the whole purpose of your explanation is to provide your patient with just as much information – no more and no less – as will allow a management plan acceptable to both of you to emerge.

Options and choice

It is human nature never to be satisfied. We seldom seem to have just the right amount of choice. Too little, and we feel powerless and resentful; too much, and we dither and become paralysed with indecision. Nevertheless, if choice is good (or so goes the mantra of the consumer society), more choice must be better. Take, for example, the matter of choosing a new car. Gone are the days of Henry Ford, when the customer could have any colour as long as it was black. There is now such a bewildering array of makes, models and specifications that we are liable to end up making a choice for non-rational reasons, such as brand loyalty, the seductiveness of the advertising, the personality of the salesman or the toss of a coin.

General practice is probably the field of medicine where there is maximum uncertainty about what is the 'right' thing to do, and hence the greatest potential for there to be acceptable alternative options. In many everyday situations, evidence about best management is sketchy, inconclusive or non-existent. Clinical guidelines, tempting though it is to regard them as dogma, are only suggestions, not intended to apply in every case.

Some of the problems presented to the GP are so minor that, frankly, it doesn't matter what treatment is given. It really doesn't matter whether a parent treats a child's common cold with Calpol®, simple linctus, homeopathic aconite or nothing at all – apart, that is, from the danger of reinforcing inappropriate health beliefs. At the opposite end of the seriousness spectrum, some situations allow only one acceptable course of action. If you make a tentative diagnosis of ruptured ectopic pregnancy, there is only one thing to do – arrange immediate hospital admission; and if this were an SCA case, you would fail the station if you did anything else. It is in the middle ground that most difficulties arise, where genuine alternative options exist and where it is possible for you and the patient to have different preferences.

What choices should you offer?

It would be foolish, and a hostage to fortune, to invite the patient to consider an option you couldn't live with if you had to. And you should certainly put forward, though not necessarily *first*, your own preferred suggestion – 'Plan A.' You might also mention any clinically acceptable alternatives. It is possible, too, that the patient has already given you some indication of their own ideas or expectations, which you should mention in language or tone of voice that indicates you are taking them seriously.

So to David Wren, you might say something like, 'I'd like to get some blood tests done to check on the *H. pylori* possibility, and then see you again. And maybe your wife would like to come as well? In the meantime, you could either continue with the indigestion tablets you've been buying or I could prescribe some more powerful antacid tablets, called omeprazole.' Given my personal background in conventional medicine, I would *not* say to him, 'Other options would be for you to consult an iridologist or a faith healer,' theoretical possibilities though they be.

How much choice does your patient want?

Some patients are happy – perhaps unhealthily so – simply to have you tell them what to do. Nonetheless, I suggest you should still let them know the various options you have considered before making your recommendation. Increasingly common, however, is the patient who has consulted Doctor Google and is therefore already aware of, but not necessarily well-informed about, a wide range of possible solutions to their problem. Some of these will be realistic, others fanciful. It may be that you will need to trim the list of options to manageable proportions.

The clearer your sense of a patient's health beliefs and expectations, the easier it is to tell how much involvement they might like in the decision-making, and to calibrate your option-giving accordingly. One patient, for example, might say, 'You see so much in the papers, on TV, it's all very confusing. So I'd rather find out what *you* thought I should do.' Another might say, 'My friend who had the same problem just got given some cream, which didn't work. So I thought, there must be other things I could try.' Ask yourself: for which of these two is the 'options and choice' agenda more appropriate?

If you misjudge a patient's desire for choice, the conversation can become almost farcical. 'We could do A, B or C. Which would you prefer?' *'I don't know. You're the doctor, you tell me.'* 'No no, you're the patient, *you* tell me.' *'No no …'* One way to avoid this game of word-tennis is to say something like, 'I don't know whether you'd thought of any of the ways we could proceed …?' The patient's response will give you a steer as to how explicit you need to be about the possibilities. Another way is to say, out loud, the dilemma you are in: 'I'm not sure whether you'd like me to run through the various ways we could tackle this, or if you'd prefer me just to tell you what I think we should do.' Here again, the patient's reply will resolve the difficulty.

Choice or the illusion of choice?

For choice to be meaningful, the options have to be realistic. To offer your patient a choice of X or Y where you know Y is unacceptable is no choice at all. Neither is creating Y for no other reason than to give the *illusion* of choice. To say to the patient with suspected ectopic pregnancy – and I'm sure you wouldn't – 'I could get you into hospital, or we could just see how things go' would be unprofessional at every level.

That is an extreme example of a spurious choice. More plausible is the way it is possible, through the use of value-laden language, to exert subtle pressure on a patient to choose the option we ourselves favour. Suppose a patient has a small skin tag that you could tie off or diathermy in seconds. But no, the patient has private health insurance and wants to 'see the finest man in Harley Street.' Might you not be tempted to say, 'Yes of course, I can refer you to Mr Hackitoff up at Saint Slashers, and hope he's having one of his sober days. Or we could easily take care of it here, where you already know everybody?' Again, I exaggerate; but might you not say to the antibiotic-seeking mother of a child with a cold, 'I could certainly give you a prescription for amoxicillin. I'll also prescribe something for diarrhoea, because you'll almost certainly need it. But I'd have thought that, as a sensible parent, you'd rather take the healthier option …?'

Whether this admittedly manipulative use of language is ethically justified is for you to decide. But we should be aware of just how sensitive our patients are, when invited to choose between options, to the nuances of how we present them.

Shared decision-making

Rather like *IdeasConcernsandExpectations*, 'shared decision-making' has become something of a cliché in the vocabulary of the consultation, a catchphrase easy to rattle off in theoretical discussion but not so easy to implement in real life. Do you believe in your patient making a significant contribution to planning the management of their problem? Of course you do; how could you *not*? Do you try to put this principle into action? Of course you do, mostly, on a good day. Is sharing the decision-making a routine part of your normal consulting style? Errmm …

It is in cultivating a cooperative approach to management that many of us find it hardest to let go of the 'Doctor knows best, so Doctor decides' legacy of the medical model we were trained in. Learning new factual knowledge or technical skills is comparatively easy; updating our attitudes and values and getting into the habit of expressing them in behaviour is much more difficult. It's not surprising that, as with many complex skills, our early attempts can seem clumsy or half-hearted. It is not sufficient, having delivered a doctor-centred statement of what needs to be done, just to tack on 'Do you have any questions?' or 'Is that OK?' and think that, with that simple formula, you have somehow turned a directive into a collaboration.

In my book *The Inner Consultation*[12] I suggested that the third of five successive 'checkpoints' to reach in the course of the consultation was 'Handover,' by which I meant making sure that the patient is happy with, and committed to, whatever management plan was decided. Chapter B3 of that book contains an excellent account,[13] in more detail than is appropriate here, of various consulting skills that can help to build the necessary sense of partnership, including:

- *Negotiating:* Have a starting position – 'Plan A' – by all means. But be prepared to consider alternative suggestions and make compromises if you can do so without jeopardising the patient's safety. Don't go too far with one particular idea without checking to see what the patient thinks about it.

- *Influencing:* State the pros and cons of the various options, but without manipulatively trying to force a particular outcome. Correct any misunderstandings the patient may have, but without antagonising or belittling them.

- *Pacing:* Things that may seem obvious to you, and hence can be stated quickly, may take a little while to be understood and considered by the patient. Allow time for what you are saying to sink in, and give the patient the opportunity to ask questions as you go along.

- *'Gift-wrapping':* Just as you would wrap a birthday gift in nice paper, accompanied by a hand-written card, in order to give the recipient maximum pleasure, you should do your best to present your management suggestions in as kind and personalised a way as possible.

When we were considering the Patient's part, I urged you to let the patient take the lead in the early stages of the consultation, able to say whatever they wanted to say with as little input from you as possible. As a rule of thumb, I think the opposite should be the case at the start of the Shared part; you should go first. If you don't, and if you begin by saying, 'Well, what do *you* think we should do?'—the patient is likely to be disconcerted by your apparent uncertainty, mistaking your reticence for incompetence. Patients come to you seeking help with a problem, to which end they give you a lot of information and expose themselves, figuratively and literally,

---

[12] Neighbour R. (2005). *The Inner Consultation: how to develop an effective and intuitive consulting style*, 2nd edition. Abingdon: CRC Press.

[13] Well I would say that, wouldn't I?

to your scrutiny. In exchange, as the consultation moves into its 'What-are-we-going-to-do-about-it?' phase, they feel entitled to expect you to deliver on your side of the contract and give them what they came for. You need to give the patient something to respond to. Unless, early on, you reveal at least something of your own analysis and proposals, the consultation risks degenerating into a game of *'Guess what I'm thinking.'*

I don't want to give any more specific advice on how to involve your patient in decision-making, because formulaic 'doing it by the book' is the antithesis of what is required. This part of the consultation should ideally be a free-flowing exchange of ideas between two people aiming to find common ground.

Nevertheless, there is one strategy that pulls together most of what is important in the previous sections; namely, for you to do your own thinking about how to manage the problem *out loud*, so that the patient can hear the way your mind is working. Thinking aloud:

- is an authentic way of genuinely involving the patient;
- can help overcome numerous problems and difficulties in the consultation;
- ensures that the decision-making is not only shared but *felt* to be shared.

Thinking aloud

Do you remember, back in your school days, learning arithmetic and being taught how to do long division? Probably you were given some sums to do for homework – divide 1,260,259 by 37, for example (Figure 4.17).

Long division: Divide 1260259 by 37, showing your working

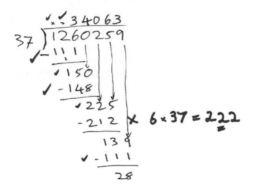

FIGURE 4.17

Almost certainly, you were told to 'show your working,' so that the teacher could follow the process you went through in doing the calculation and, if you made a mistake, could see where you went wrong and help you with whichever step needed a bit of extra attention.

By the same token, if you begin the Shared part of the consultation by thinking aloud so that the patient can follow the workings of your own mind, you give the patient the best possible chance of being genuinely involved in planning the management.

As you draw a line under the data-gathering part of the consultation, knowing that the next thing will be to open up a discussion of possible ways forward, you will be silently weighing up a number of factors that all have a bearing on what plan is finally agreed. These include:

- your provisional diagnosis or assessment of the patient's problem and the issues it raises;
- the 'Plan A' that is your own preferred option;
- any realistic alternative options and their pros and cons;
- the possible consequences of the various options;
- what you think are the patient's own expectations, priorities and preferences;
- anything you feel you absolutely *must* do;
- anything you absolutely *can't or won't* do;
- your own dilemmas or areas of uncertainty;
- any practical constraints on your freedom of action, e.g. clinical guidelines, referral or prescribing policies, waiting lists; and
- any points where you would genuinely like guidance or an opinion from the patient.

A key word in the previous paragraph is *silently*. Much of our problem analysis and decision-planning takes place behind closed lips, in the secret domain of our private thoughts, to which we allow the patient only limited access. We are often reluctant to let the patient see the workings of our professional mind, even though he or she has a major stake in the outcome of our silent deliberations. The reasons for this reluctance are varied. Some of our thought processes can seem to us so obvious as to be taken for granted. It just never occurs to us that the patient might be interested in following them. But sometimes we keep our thoughts to ourselves for more questionable reasons. We might be unsure of how to proceed and embarrassed to reveal our indecision or lack of knowledge. We might be afraid the patient will become challenging or hostile. Sometimes we want to steer the patient towards a particular course of action, but don't want to be caught doing so. Let's be honest – it is not just the patient who sometimes has a hidden agenda for the consultation; we quite often do the same.

There is no need to be so shy about letting the patient in on your thoughts. I want to encourage you to be more forthcoming – indeed, to be quite explicit – about what is in your mind as you begin the Shared part of the consultation. Spell it out and let the patient respond. Cast aside the mask of professional inscrutability. Put your cards on the table and see which one the patient picks up. This strategy of frank self-disclosure may at first sound risky, putting yourself in an unnecessarily vulnerable position. But it has real advantages, as we shall see shortly. If your assessment and your ideas about management make sense to *you*, they ought to make sense to the patient. (And if they don't make sense to the patient, maybe they aren't quite so sensible!) Moreover, if you have any hidden agenda but don't disclose it, the results can be as disruptive as when a patient does it to *you*.

Think back to the example of the arithmetic homework: if you don't show your working, the teacher can only mark your answer *right* or *wrong*. This is of limited educational value. If you got the sum right, it may well be because you completely understand what you're doing. But it could just have been a fluke, or two errors cancelling themselves out. If you were incorrect, you won't know where you went wrong. Even if the teacher tells you that the correct answer is in fact 34,061, remainder 2, that information alone is unhelpful unless you can see at what point your own calculation deviated from the process that would have led to it. But if you *do* show your working, the teacher knows where to target their future input for maximum helpfulness.

To take this analogy into the clinical situation: hearing you present the full range of your thoughts gives the patient something useful to respond to. He or she is free to pick up on whatever point is most relevant or most in need of further discussion. A conversation that begins, in effect, with you saying, 'Let me tell you everything I'm thinking …,' to which the patient can reply, 'Let's talk more about this particular point…' is likely to focus quickly and productively on exactly that aspect of management where the decision-making most needs to be shared. And what the patient wants to discuss may not be what you were expecting or hoping.

To make this idea more concrete, let's pick up the consultation with David Wren as it reaches the Shared part. If you keep your thoughts to yourself, what will he see? He will see you pause, obviously thinking, and he might then hear you say, 'Hmmm … Right. I think you've probably got an infection called *H. pylori*, and I'd like to do some tests for that.

I don't think you need referral to a specialist. Is that OK?' That may or may not be a good plan, but how is Mr Wren to judge? Without knowing how you reached that conclusion – what was in your mind when you went *Hmmm* –, how is he to know whether he can trust your judgement, or what alternatives you've considered, or whether any of your plan is negotiable?

Imagine instead that you were to say something like this:

> Mr Wren, let me tell you what my thoughts are at the moment? On the strength of what I've learned from you today, I can be pretty sure you don't have cancer. Probably 99% sure. It's much more likely – *much* more likely – that you have an infection with a germ called *H. pylori*. It causes symptoms like yours, it's quite common, and it's easy to treat with antibiotics, so I'd like to do a test for that. Or it could just be that your stomach is making too much acid. But I do understand how worried you and your wife are about the cancer possibility. The only way to be 100% sure would be for me to send you to the hospital, either to see a specialist or to have an endoscopy – that's where they put an inspection tube down into your stomach. It's not very pleasant, and many doctors would think it was unnecessary in view of your mild symptoms. But it might just be the only way to put your or your wife's mind at rest. I'm not sure what's the best thing. What do you think?

Admittedly, that is quite a long speech. But it captures as succinctly as possible the various factors you are having to weigh up. Put yourself in Mr Wren's position as he hears you put your thoughts into words, and imagine how he might respond. Which particular part of your 'thinking aloud' he picks up on will depend on his own priorities: how anxious he is, or his wife; how reassured he is by your '99%' confidence; what the magazine article said; how much he knows, or wants to know, about *H. pylori*; what he feels about drugs or hospitals or specialists; or whether he has something else in mind that you haven't even considered.

Suppose he says to you, 'So you don't think I've got cancer. That'll be a load off my mind, and my wife's as well. The article we read also mentioned this infection thing – could you tell me more about that?' It's clear from his reply how *this* Mr Wren – let's call him 'Mr Wren #1' – wants the management-planning discussion to proceed. He is happy with your '99% reassurance,' and expects that his wife will be also. So you don't need to say anything more at this stage about referrals or endoscopies. Instead, you can tell him about *Helicobacter* and how you will test for it. He has indicated (and I'm sure you have appreciated) that the views of his wife, although she is not present today, have to be considered. So you will probably suggest that she attend with him when he comes back for the test results. You might want to offer him a leaflet, if you have one, about dyspepsia to take home and read together, possibly as a counterweight to the magazine article that has triggered the anxiety. But (you will tell him), he must consult you promptly if he develops any so-called red flag symptoms such as vomiting of blood, worsening pain or weight loss. Mr Wren #1 has not asked about any other measures to relieve his symptoms. So here again, you could think aloud: 'I could give you some more effective antacid tablets if you like'; and his reply will let you know whether or not to prescribe, say, a proton pump inhibitor.

The consultation with Mr Wren #1 is now almost done. Within a few minutes, the discussion prompted by your thinking aloud will have led to a management plan acceptable to you both: give him relevant factual information, test for the most likely diagnosis, book an early review appointment with him and his wife. Mr Wren #1 will leave the room less anxious than he entered it, knowing that he is in safe hands, that he has been taken seriously and his point of view is respected, and with a clear idea of what to say to his wife. You also can be satisfied with the outcome; it is, after all, very close to your original Plan A. Your patient is safe; your management is clinically sound and tailored to the patient's specific concerns and expectations. Job done.

Another Mr Wren, Mr Wren #2, might respond to your 'thinking aloud' speech quite differently. He's a pessimist. 'You're telling me I *could* have cancer,' he says. 'One in a hundred? It'll be me; I know it will. So yes, please, I want to see a specialist, get this tube thing done as soon as possible. Neither of us will get a wink of sleep until I know for sure.'

The conversation that follows will be very different from that with Mr Wren #1; and it is not what you were hoping for. You might want to check what he is telling you: 'So you would like me to organise a hospital referral …?' But if he confirms that this is indeed what he wants – well, at least you know your agenda for the rest of this consultation. Even though you may face a struggle with the clinical guidelines and referral protocols, you know you will have to brace yourself for it because nothing else is going to satisfy Mr Wren #2. You'll explain how the referral process works, probably invoking the 'fast track for suspected cancer.' You'll arrange routine blood tests and possibly an *H. pylori* test, 'because the specialist will expect these to have been done before they see you.' And you will still offer to see him again with his wife, not only because it is good practice to include her in the management but also because an early follow-up appointment with them might give them the opportunity to change their minds about the referral.

It is of course open to you, after Mr Wren #2's initial response, to think aloud some more: 'I was rather hoping you wouldn't say that, because it will be quite difficult to arrange, and I'd prefer to rule out the more likely causes of your symptoms first.' But there is a danger that, if you try too hard to (as he will see it) fob him off, he will continue to present with worsening symptoms, or will consult another doctor whom he hopes will be more compliant, or will return with his wife in a confrontational mood. Situations like this, where you and the patient have strong preferences for different management options, also raise an important ethical issue: where do your loyalties lie – to the wishes of the individual patient, to your own interpretation of best practice, or to the good husbandry of National Health Service resources? My personal opinion is that if, as we often claim, a GP's role is to be the patient's advocate, and if the idea of shared management is to be more than empty words, then we owe a greater responsibility to the patient than to the State. But (as they say) 'other views are available.'

Now imagine how a third Mr Wren might reply to your 'thinking aloud' speech. Mr Wren #3, luckily, is less challenging than #2. He says, 'You're the doctor. I'll do whatever you think is best.' With Mr Wren #3, you can now be doctor-centred with a clear conscience. His decision is that you should decide. For you to take responsibility *is* to be patient-centred. So you proceed: 'OK, let's get the blood and *Helicobacter* tests organised and see you and your wife together in a week's time. Also … a leaflet … prescribe a PPI tablet … red flag symptoms … any questions?' He will leave satisfied, and again, so can you be – your patient is safe, your clinical management is sound and safety-netted, and the decision-making has been as fully shared as the patient wanted.

Mr Wren #4 says, 'As for me, I'm happy to get the tests done that you advise and see what they show. But my wife, she's a real worrier, and in this article, it said about getting an endoscopy.' This response shows you need to spend the next few minutes planning the reassurance of the absent Mrs Wren #4. How could you do this? You could invite her to make an appointment for herself; or come with her husband; or you could telephone her to explain what is happening; or you could give her a copy of the (increasingly essential) leaflet; or you could rehearse with Mr Wren what he is to say to her when he gets home. Which would be best? Think aloud. Say to Mr Wren #4, 'I'd like to put your wife in the picture. I can give you a leaflet for her to read, and then she could come and see me, either on her own or with you. Or I could give her a call. What would be best from her point of view, do you think?' And Mr Wren will tell you. If you share your uncertainty with him, he will tell you.

Other versions of Mr Wren are also possible, each listening to your 'thinking aloud' speech. The response of each 'Mr Wren' will give you the starting point you need in order for the subsequent discussion to be as relevant as possible to the individual patient. Thus:

Mr Wren #5: 'I don't care what we do as long as I don't have to go to hospital.'

You: 'OK, we'll arrange some tests here, and I'll try you on a stronger antacid tablet and see you again in two weeks. But if your symptoms get worse or the tests show anything unexpected, we might have to re-think the "no hospital" plan.'

Mr Wren #6: 'Can't I just carry on with the antacid tablets, and cut down on smoking and drinking?'

You: 'Indeed you can; and if you'd like some help with the smoking and drinking, our nurse runs a very useful clinic which you could come to. But … red flags … follow-up … perhaps come with your wife.'

Mr Wren #7: 'Could it just be stress?'

You: 'Yes, it could. What would you say are the main sources of stress in your life?' *(Further brief discussion.)* 'Why don't we get some basic tests done, to make sure we're not missing anything serious; then, when you come again, we can talk about stress and what you could do about it.'

I hope you can see the common thread in all these examples. Think it, say it, discuss it (Figure 4.18). When you think aloud, giving the patient a window into your own thought processes, the patient's response carries you straight to the heart of what matters most to that individual patient. To my mind, the discussion this generates results in management planning that is not only genuinely shared but is also *felt* to be shared.

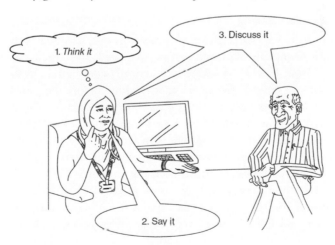

FIGURE 4.18

Have a look back at the beginning of this section, where I marked off the first two paragraphs from [A] to [B]. That passage was my attempt to put into words the various thoughts I was having at the time I wrote it. Now imagine that I am here in the room with you and that I say those words out loud and ask you to respond. How do you think you might reply? You might say, 'Just get on with it!' or 'My problem is, I always seem to run out of time for management planning,' or 'When I try to share the decision-making, I sound very unsure of myself.' Whatever your reply, it would help me focus on your own personal expectations instead of (as I must do in print) just having to guess and hope for the best.

Signpost your thinking aloud

It's a good idea to preface your thinking aloud with a few words that let the patient know what's going on. The time has come, after all, when the patient has to switch from being the answerer of questions in the Doctor's part to an active participant in the decision-making. You might, for instance, say something like:

> 'I'm going to tell you what my ideas are about what we could do, and then I'd like you to tell me your own thoughts,' or

> 'Let's talk about how to deal with this problem. I'll start by telling you where *I* am with it, and then perhaps you'll tell me what you think.'

Experiment with different ways of introducing your thinking aloud until you find a form of words that feels comfortable to you.

Checking for understanding

Whatever management plan you arrive at is only as good as the extent to which it is implemented, and that in turn needs the patient to understand and accept it. Hence the advice in practically every guide to the consultation that you should 'check for understanding' before the patient leaves.

This advice, like so much else, is easier to give than to carry out. Patients are often anxious to please, and will sometimes give the appearance of understanding while the opposite is in fact the case. A perfunctory 'Any questions?' is likely to result in an equally half-hearted 'No, that's fine,' after which, collusion of satisfaction, the patient will depart in a state of bewildered non-compliance. A common gimmick is to ask the patient, 'What will you tell your wife/husband/partner about today's consultation when you get home?' Apart from being an irritating cliché, this formula can lead to embarrassment if the patient has no partner, or for some reason, wants to keep the contents of your discussion private.

Another even more annoying tactic is to ask the patient to summarise back to you the key points and outcome of the consultation. It is almost impossible for this to sound anything other than patronising and school-teacher-y. Patients hate it.

If you pay close attention to your patient's facial expression, tone of voice and body language, your everyday sensitivity to social cues will usually suggest what, if anything, the patient is having difficulty with. If you're not sure, you could try asking, 'Is this making sense? Is there anything I'm saying that you'd like me to go over again?'

By all means, ask the patient if they have any questions. But do so in a concerned and permissive manner. Give them time to think and to answer, and to tell you what aspect they would like to be further explained. An offer to write down important details or of an explanatory diagram or a relevant information leaflet might be appreciated. (But don't overdo the freehand drawings unless you really are a second Leonardo da Vinci.)

Safety-netting

I introduced the concept of safety-netting in my 1987 book *The Inner Consultation*, and it has now become a recognised component of good practice. In general practice, uncertainty is a fact of life, and the unexpected is always just around the corner. Safety-netting is the advance contingency planning that will keep you and the patient safe in unforeseen circumstances. In principle, safety-netting consists of asking yourself the following three questions, and before the patient leaves the room, you should know the answers to all of them:

1   If the management plan works out, what do I expect to happen?
2   How would the patient or I know if things didn't go as expected?
3   In that case, what would we do next?

The stock phrase of the caricature GP is in fact an excellent example of safety-netting: 'Take two paracetamol, and call me in the morning if it's not better.' A more realistic example would be if you were to say to a patient, 'The tablets should help your painful knee – try them for two weeks. But if they don't seem to be working, come and see me again. And make an urgent appointment if the knee ever gets hot and swollen.' Or (to Mr Wren), 'If the tests for *H. pylori* come back negative, and if the omeprazole doesn't help, then I would probably want to refer you for a specialist opinion.'

The specific details of your safety-netting will obviously depend on the nature of the problem you are dealing with. And it is a matter of judgement as to how explicit you will be in spelling out your 'what if?' thoughts to the patient. Safety-netting is not a prescribed set of actions or remarks; it's more a precautionary attitude of mind. It is always good practice to think one step ahead of events.

Closing the consultation

The final moments of the consultation provide an opportunity, if you need one, to recap its key points – the diagnosis, the management plan, what the patient is to do next and the follow-up arrangements.

That done, most consultations will end as they began, with an exchange of civilities: 'Nice to see you,' 'I hope that's been helpful,' 'Mind how you go.' Such remarks are the conversational equivalent of an after-dinner mint. They give a gentle signal that the consultation is over and it is time for the patient to leave, hopefully on a note of mutual regard that further cements the ongoing relationship between you.

Some doctors – though it can seem like asking for trouble – like to enquire, expecting the answer *No*, 'Was there anything else I can do for you today?' They have perhaps learned the hard way that sometimes a patient, realising time is almost up, will at the last minute feel emboldened to raise a fresh, significant issue. Irritating though this can be, it is important to remain alert to any verbal or non-verbal cues that the patient may have some further undisclosed agenda. We will return to the challenges posed by the 'While I'm here' patient in the next section.

Nevertheless, it is useful to have up one's sleeve a few unobtrusive ways of, shall we say, 'speeding the parting guest.'

- A brief summary, delivered with a note of finality, of the consultation's main points and conclusions sends a clear message, e.g. 'So, if we just sum up …'
- Firmer still would be, 'Well, I think we've taken that as far as we can for now …,' or 'I'm afraid that has to be the end of our time for today. But please make another appointment if you'd like to.'
- In the days when prescriptions were usually handwritten, the 'thwipp' of a script being torn from the pad carried a suggestion of dismissal that the soft whirring of a laser printer cannot replicate. However, to be handed a prescription, leaflet or appointment card can still feel like being given 'something to be going home with.'
- We saw how, in the Patient's part, various non-verbal factors help to build rapport and encourage the patient to talk, such as: a 'Goldilocks' physical distance between your chairs, neither too close nor too far apart; a comfortable degree of eye contact; an open body posture. It

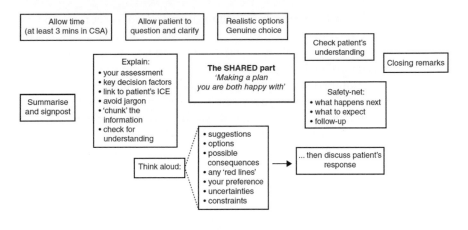

FIGURE 4.19

is possible to convey the opposite message by reversing these rapport-building measures. Thus, moving your chair away from (or even closer to) the patient, reducing the amount of eye contact, or turning away and closing your body posture all send subliminal signals that communication is coming to an end.

In real life, closure is seldom difficult if you have identified the right problem, agreed on a course of action that satisfies the patient's concerns and priorities and made sure the patient understands what is going on and what happens next. There should be no need for you to go as far as a friend of mine, a highly respected contributor to the consultation literature, who claims that *in extremis*, faced with a patient who seems settled in for the night, his tactic of last resort is to start to change into a tuxedo.

In the SCA, the examiner will stop marking your consultation on the stroke of 12 minutes, whether or not you have completed it. Nonetheless, it can only help you gain marks under 'Relating to others' if, within that time, you can round the consultation off nicely, perhaps with a brief recap of what has been agreed, and a few friendly or encouraging words.

Figure 4.19 summarises the ingredients of a successful Shared part.

More about thinking aloud

I have advocated thinking aloud – telling the patient what is going through your mind – as an effective way of kick-starting the decision-sharing stage of the consultation. But I want to go further than that. The same policy of openness, of self-disclosure, has much to commend it at other times and for other purposes. In fact, I want to encourage you to become a doctor who is comfortable thinking aloud as a matter of course, making it just a part of how you routinely talk to patients.

As the consultation unfolds, right from the start, there are times when we are not quite sure what to say or do next; moments when it's not clear what is going on or how to proceed. We may have a niggling sense that the consultation needs a bit of steering, some structure or some limits, or a change of focus. At such times, it would often help to have some input from the patient, to know their point of view. But how can you do it? Turning a receipt, as we discussed earlier in this book, is one way. But thinking aloud is an alternative, and sometimes a better one. If anything about what is happening in the consultation should cause you a problem, don't feel you have to stay tight-lipped; say it out loud. In effect, tell the patient what the difficulty is and ask for their help or guidance. The patient will almost always come to the rescue.

Here are some examples of how thinking aloud can be helpful in the Patient's part:

- A 60-year-old woman is telling you a rambling story of her painful knees, a mother with dementia, some tablets and a new social worker. 'Can I pause you there? I'm not sure,' you say, thinking aloud, 'whether your main concern at the moment is your arthritis or your mum's long-term care.' 'Well, the knees, I suppose,' your patient explains, 'because I'll need to be properly mobile if she has to come and live with me.' And now you have a better idea of today's agenda.

- 'I know you doctors don't like being given a long list of problems,' a 45-year-old man begins, 'but I've got a mole on my back that's started to itch, I think I'm due a blood pressure check, my wife wants her prescription, and I need some advice, because I'm pretty sure our Gavin is on drugs.' 'Oof!' you sigh. 'The problem that gives me is that of course I want to help with all those things, but if we go much over ten minutes, the other patients who are waiting will start to get cross.' 'Fair enough,' says the patient. 'Have a look at the mole first, that shouldn't take long. Then we'll see how much we've got time for.' Knowing your difficulty, the patient has prioritised his own list and will not be resentful if asked to make another appointment to talk about Gavin.

- An irate woman, a frequent attender, is complaining that another doctor in the practice 'told me my headaches were all in my mind, and I didn't need a scan. Well, I'm not having that, so I've come to see you!' You count to ten while you think how to put it tactfully: 'Some problems get everybody frustrated,' you begin, 'myself included. But I hope you won't expect me to order a scan just because my colleague didn't.' You have acknowledged the feelings of all concerned, and indicated that you are not going to be manipulated out of exercising your own clinical judgement. 'No, of course not,' she replies, 'I just felt he didn't take me seriously. Anyway, about these headaches …'

Now some examples of thinking aloud in the Doctor's part:

- 'I'd like to examine you now. I ought to offer you a chaperone, but unfortunately there doesn't seem to be anyone available at the moment.' 'That's all right, Doctor, go ahead; we know each other well enough.'
- (The patient is a woman with pelvic inflammatory disease.) 'I need to ask you a personal question, but I'm worried I might offend you.' 'That's all right, Doctor, go ahead.' 'OK. Is there any possibility your husband might have caught an infection from someone outside your marriage?' There's a long pause, and then you continue, 'You look shocked; or maybe you think I should mind my own business.' The patient begins to weep: 'I've had my suspicions …'
- Dermatology was never your strong point, and the patient has a lesion you don't recognise. You're not a good bluffer either, so you say, 'I don't know what it is. I'd like to look through my skins book and see if I can find a picture that looks like the thing on your hand.' (The last time I said this to a patient, he said, 'Can I look too?')

Patients know that when they talk to a doctor, they may be expected to disclose information that is usually kept private. If they find you willing to be frank about your own inner thoughts – difficulties, doubts and all – it makes it easier for them also to open up. The result is usually to make the conversation a more authentic meeting of adult minds and to deepen the feeling of mutual respect.

At an exam preparation course where I was a tutor, I was encouraging the would-be candidates to share some of their difficulties and uncertainties with their patients, in the belief (which I still hold) that doing so enhances rather than damages their credibility in the eyes of the patient. One of the groups challenged me. She said, 'You have to be really confident to think aloud. At our career stage, there are lots of things we're uncertain about. If we keep saying *I'm not sure about this* and *I don't know that*, it sounds a bit pathetic.' Before I could respond, another course member intervened. 'If you don't feel confident,' she said, 'pretend that you are.'

I think that is good advice. There is a sense in which general practice is a performance art, in that how you present yourself to your patient carries a message over and above your competence as a clinician. It is not enough to know your lines; you have to deliver them in such a way that your audience – your patient – finds them convincing.

Imagine yourself back consulting with Mr Wren, this time at a loss as to what appropriate management of his 'indigestion' might be. The scene could play out in two different ways. In the first, you say to him, in a timid and apologetic voice, 'Oh dear, I've not had to deal with anybody with indigestion before. I suppose I could see if there's anything in the textbook. Or Google it. Do you mind if I just pop out and ask if anyone knows what we'd normally do?' Alternatively, you could act the role – though it's not really a pretence, is it? – of a competent professional. 'Mister Wren,' you say, in a confident voice, 'I've not met this exact situation before, and I want to make sure I arrange the best treatment for you. So I'd like to discuss it with one of my more experienced colleagues.'

The same plan – ask someone else for advice – but two very different scenarios. After the first, a startled Mr Wren will probably go straight out and book another appointment with a 'proper' doctor. In the second, he can relax, knowing he is safe in your hands. Your acting confident is no confidence trick. His continuing trust in you would not be misplaced; the care you arrange will be trustworthy.

Thinking aloud is more than a technique or a strategy; it's a matter of personal style, almost a philosophy. The very fact that you are willing to open up your thought processes to scrutiny and discussion sends a message to your patients about the type of doctor you are and the way you like to do your medicine.

Decisions about what we say and do emerge from an often unconscious interplay of multiple factors: the information at our disposal; our personal goals and priorities; the options available to us and their possible consequences; our emotional state; our beliefs and values. The relationships we allow to develop with our patients have ground rules that, in part, reflect our own values.[14] Conventional medical education tends to result in the default doctor–patient relationship being an asymmetrical one, in which the doctor expects to have free access to the inner workings of the patient's mind, but not vice versa. But if we are to take seriously the notion that the consultation is 'a meeting of experts,[15] then that asymmetry has to

---

[14] This and related ideas about the clinical impact of the doctor's own psychology are further explored in my book *The Inner Physician* (CRC Press, 2016).

[15] Tuckett D. (1985). *Meetings between Experts: An Approach to Sharing Ideas in Medical Consultations*. Tavistock. Psychoanalyst David Tuckett first articulated the idea that while the doctor has medical expertise, the patient is the expert in his or her own life.

be challenged. The more two people know about how each other's mind works, the easier it is for them to reach consensus.

Anyway, thinking aloud works. It makes for more easygoing but, at the same time, more meaningful consultations. Most experienced GPs would agree that, as their careers progress, they grow increasingly comfortable with letting the patient 'see the workings.' In fact, it comes as something of a relief, rather like discovering that your friends love you just as much even if you don't always try to hold your stomach in.

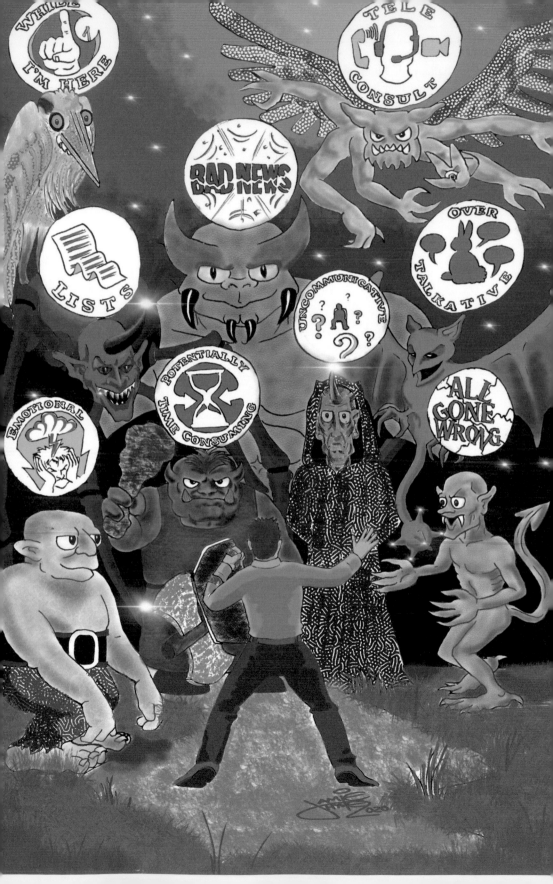

5

Some particular challenges

In this book, I'm trying to describe a way of conducting your consultations that is as generalisable as possible; in other words, one that will work in most situations. But generalisable is not the same as universal. A formulaic 'one size fits all' approach will never suit general practice, where the fact that every patient and every problem are different is both its delight and its challenge. To consult rigidly 'by the book' – *any* book – would be disrespectful to patients and unfulfilling for the doctor. The essence of professionalism is tailoring one's skills to the needs of each individual who needs them.

One of my own mentors in the 1970s was the humanistic psychologist John Heron.[1] I once heard him asked for his thoughts on what it meant to be a professional. He replied, 'A professional is someone who has a wide range of options, and can move cleanly and elegantly amongst them.' Cleanness and elegance: two features of a consulting style I hope we would all aspire to. The Italians have a word for it: *sprezzatura*, which means nimbleness under pressure, apparently effortless flexibility, making what is difficult look easy. I make no claim that this book will endow anyone with *sprezzatura*; but I do believe one's consultations should have a solid foundation of structure and skill on which to make elegant personalised variations.

Key principles to take forward from what you have already read are:

- Try to understand the problem from the patient's point of view.
- It's okay – indeed, it's necessary – sometimes to 'steer' the consultation in order to achieve the most benefit in the time available.

---

[1] John Heron, b 1928, was an Assistant Director of the British Postgraduate Medical Federation and Director of the Human Potential Research Project, University of Surrey. He developed a method of counselling called six-category intervention analysis.

This chapter begins by reminding you of a handful of techniques that will prove useful in most tricky situations. After that come some suggestions for dealing with various specific challenges all too familiar in general practice. Obviously, I can't cover every possible eventuality, but I'm sure you'll be able to grasp the principles involved and apply them in your own individual circumstances. There are also some hints on consulting by telephone or video.

Finally, I'll offer some personal advice to anyone actively preparing for the SCA.

Four things that will get you out of most difficulties

(1) Process awareness

By 'process awareness' I mean the ability, while the consultation is in full flow, to disconnect part of your attention, take a mental step back, and notice how the consultation is going – whether it is on track, or in danger of veering off course, or if anything unhelpful seems to be developing (Figure 5.1). It's being able to recognise and interpret what is going on between you and the patient while it's actually happening, so that you can make adjustments if necessary.

If you were to watch one of your consultations on video, you would probably find yourself thinking things like *You're talking too much*, or *I think there's more to this problem than you're being told*, or *You're taking too long over this – get a*

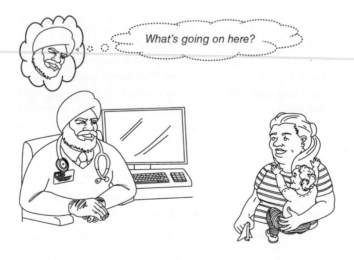

FIGURE 5.1

move on, or *Ask more open questions!* or *I don't think the patient understood that*, or *Careful – you're getting irritated, and that's how mistakes get made.* This kind of commentary can be a useful learning tool after the consultation has finished. But it's much more useful if, by developing process awareness, you can make these observations silently, 'in your mind's ear,' in real time, while the consultation is actually in progress. That way, you can do something about them.

Process awareness – mentally taking stock – is a useful response when things start to go wrong or if you are finding a consultation difficult without being quite sure why. Our subconscious mind is very good at detecting the early warning signs of an incipient problem, before our conscious mind can say exactly what the problem is. At such moments, our first inkling often comes in the form of an emotional reaction, such as a slight feeling of frustration or irritation or bewilderment – moments when something inside us seems to go 'uh-uh.' As you gain experience, you'll get better at recognising these 'uh-uh' moments and using them as a cue to pause and think *Hold on, what's going on here?*

(2) The three-part structure (Figure 5.2)

Get the patient's version of the situation as fully as you can first before you start to massage it into a form you can do medicine on. Make sure the problem you identify is the right one, i.e. the one where some help from you will bring the most benefit to the patient. And when it comes to the Shared part, remember the key message is 'Discuss, don't tell.'

Most consultations that go wrong do so for one or more of these reasons:

- The Patient's part has been skimped, usually in an attempt to save time, so that the 'right' problem has not been addressed.
- The doctor has flipped backwards and forwards between the Patient's part and the Doctor's part, resulting in 'premature medicalisation.'
- In the Shared part, only lip service has been paid to involving the patient in the decision-making.

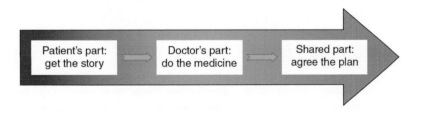

Patient's part: get the story → Doctor's part: do the medicine → Shared part: agree the plan

FIGURE 5.2

If you realise that a consultation is starting to suffer for lack of coherent structure – pause; ask yourself, *Which part of the consultation should I be in?*; then, once you're clear about that, resume in the right part, rewinding if necessary.

(3) 'Steering'

It is in everybody's interest for the consultation to stay on track and to keep within whatever time constraints apply, and it is primarily your responsibility to try and make sure it does. This means having the ability, the confidence and the resolve to steer the consultation process if necessary. Ways of doing this include:

- *Signposting:* telling the patient what's coming next, e.g. 'Now I'd like to ask you about your family history.'

- *Suggesting:* dropping a clear hint as to what you'd like to happen next e.g. 'I think we could move on now,' or 'Maybe you have some questions.'

- *Turning a receipt (the two-part steer):* acknowledging something important the patient has told you, then following up with your own agenda e.g. 'Thank you for telling me that. Before we go on, could I just check what medication you're taking?'

- *Summarising:* recapping the story so far and checking if the patient agrees, e.g. 'So, just to make sure I've understood correctly …'

- *Checking:* making sure the patient doesn't have any undeclared agenda, e.g. 'Is there anything else we haven't covered so far that you think I need to know about?'

- *Thinking aloud:* telling the patient the thoughts behind your opinion or suggestions, e.g. 'Can I tell you how this problem looks to me?'

(4) Thinking aloud

We discussed this at length a few pages ago, but thinking aloud is possibly the closest thing in the consulting skills repertoire to a master key for getting out of trouble. When in difficulty, find a tactful and non-confrontational way of explaining your difficulty to the patient, and invite them to help you solve it. Usually, they will. Think it, say it, discuss it.

The patient with a list

It is increasingly common, as rising demand threatens to outstrip the capacity of the general practice workforce, for patients to bring multiple problems to a single appointment. Often, they will organise their agenda into a written or mental list, perhaps in response to the advice to do so that some practices display. (The stern notices to be found in some waiting rooms to the effect that 'one appointment is for one problem' are generally ineffective and, in my opinion, rude.) It is not the patient's fault that they have several problems or that you are busy. By making a list, they are trying to be helpful.

Scenario

The patient is a woman in her late forties. Reading from a note that she produces from her handbag, she tells you, 'My periods seem to be getting much heavier, and sometimes I'm flooding. I could do with some more sleeping pills, only this time could you give me twice as many, because I'm finding I need them more often? And I think I'm due for my blood pressure check. Oh, and I need a letter from you for the housing, about the damp.'

The problems

There is far more here than can be competently dealt with in a single appointment, even if you are prepared to let it overrun by a few minutes. Menorrhagia is a symptom of several conditions, not all of which are benign. The insomnia may indicate depression, something which ideally you would like to explore. The blood pressure check could be done by a nurse; but then, it probably would only take you a minute. Writing letters to Local Authority housing departments, you know from experience, is tedious and usually futile. The effect of this lengthy agenda and its implications is to produce in you a heart-sink reaction that may carry over and contaminate your dealings with subsequent patients.

In the case scenario, the patient has revealed her full list at the outset. But it would have been more problematic had she begun, 'I've got several things to discuss. First, my periods …,' without mentioning what else was on the list, or, worse, waited until you had spent 7 minutes dealing with the menorrhagia before saying, 'Anyway, that was the first thing. Next, I need some extra sleeping pills.'

What needs to happen

For this to be a tolerably successful consultation, you need to know the patient's complete agenda; the earlier the better. Then you need to prioritise it, making sure that you deal with what is medically urgent and/or the patient's top priority, while making contingency plans for the likelihood that you will have to defer some items for a subsequent consultation.

You might also want (in a sinister-sounding phrase coined by Stott and Davis[2]) to 'modify her help-seeking behaviour'; in other words, to suggest

---

[2] Stott NCH and Davis RH. (1979). The exceptional potential in each primary care consultation. J R Coll Gen Pract. 29:201–205.

better ways of using the healthcare system. Specifically, if in future she has several problems, she might consider booking a double appointment, the practice nurse could do the blood pressure check and perhaps she could let you have a written summary of the points she would like you to make to the housing department.

Not least, you would like the consultation not to wreck your own composure and leave you flustered or bad-tempered for the next patient you see.

How you can make it happen

The patient who produces a written list makes things easy for you, particularly if (with a two-part steer) you can say, 'Thank you, that's helpful. Would you mind if I take a look at it?' Not only does physical possession of the list symbolically give you a measure of control, but it also helps with prioritising and time management.[3]

But not all bearers of a list are so forthcoming, and you may have to rely on verbal or non-verbal cues to alert you to its existence. In the consultation's opening moments, keep your ears and eyes open for words like 'first' and 'to start with,' or for some apparent hesitation in settling on an opening account of a problem. There is a difference between a patient who says straightforwardly, 'I've come to see you about my periods,' and one who says, 'I've come to see you about … ermm … my periods; yes, that's the main thing.' It may be tempting to ignore this hint, but the list, if there is one, will not go away, and it is better to establish the fact in the first minute or two rather than much later in the consultation. If you are told, or if you suspect, that the patient is bringing several problems, I think it is acceptable, in the interests of the consultation's overall effectiveness, to compromise on the general principle of not interrupting the patient's opening narrative, in order to find out one way or another. You could do this with a two-part steer: 'You said your periods were the main thing,' *(receipt)*, 'but please tell me briefly what else you'd like to discuss today.' Or you could think aloud: 'I get the feeling there are several things you want to talk about, in which case I'd find it helpful to know at this stage rather than towards the end of our time today.'

Receipts and thinking aloud are also useful techniques for achieving your other 'process goals.' To prioritise the items on the list, for instance, you could again use a two-part steer: 'Those are all good reasons for coming. Which do you feel is the most important?' Or you could think aloud: 'I'd like to help with all those, of course, but the problem with your periods sounds perhaps

---

[3] I once had a patient who always brought a written list. On one occasion, I leaned forward and took it from him, thinking *He who holds the list holds the power.* 'I thought you might do that,' he said. He reached into his jacket pocket and produced another piece of paper, 'So I made a copy.'

the most important, medically speaking. I was also wondering whether the poor sleep might be because you were depressed. What do you think?'

Thinking aloud would be an effective way of conveying the possibility that there might not be time to cover everything in one appointment: 'It's important that we look into the reasons for your heavy periods. And I can certainly repeat your sleeping pill prescription. But if you'd like to talk some more about why you might not be sleeping, that might need more time than we're going to have today.'

Turning receipts is a good way of 'modifying help-seeking behaviour.' 'That's quite a list! Maybe another time, if you've got several things to discuss, it would be a good idea to book a double appointment.' Or, 'Yes, your blood pressure check is due. Did you know you can go to our practice nurse's clinic for that?' Or, 'You mentioned you need a housing letter for the Council. Rather than take time with that now, I'd like you to make a note of the various points you'd like me to include, and leave it with the receptionist for me, for when I do the letter.'

Patients with lists can unwittingly be very stressful for a time-pressured GP. A judicious and tactful piece of thinking aloud can provide a valuable safety valve by letting the patient appreciate that we too have our human frailties. On a particularly bad day, I have had some success by saying something along the lines of, 'You probably saw my face fall when you brought out your list of problems. It's not that I'm not interested or unwilling to help. It's just that there never seems to be enough time to do justice to what patients, quite reasonably, expect.' No patient will ever reply 'That's *your* problem.' And the expression of sympathy that followed made *me* feel better.

'While I'm here, Doctor …'

At least the patient who brings a list, provided you find out what's on it at an early stage, gives you a chance to time-manage the consultation. More challenging is the patient who, having given no hint of a problem other than the one you have been discussing for the first 8 minutes, says, 'While I'm here, can I ask you about something else?' or, 'Anyway, that was the first thing …'

Late-breaking news like this is potentially more disruptive and more likely to irritate you than a clearly flagged agenda set out in a list. It may be a genuine afterthought, easily dealt with or deferred. But equally, the patient may have kept the *While I'm here* problem deliberately concealed for an understandable reason. Perhaps it is embarrassing or a cause of serious anxiety. The first problem may have been the so-called ticket of admission, which the patient presented to see how you handled it before feeling emboldened enough to raise the second, more important issue.

The combination of a potentially important problem and you finding yourself under unanticipated time pressure results in a situation where it is easy to make an error of judgement.

Scenario #1

Your patient is a woman of 29 who has consulted you about worsening migraines. You are in the final stages of planning a change of treatment when she says, 'While I've got you – I'm starting to get pain in my back when I come off the treadmill at the gym. Would you mind having a look?'

What needs to happen?

You have three options: (1) Begin a whole new consultation about the back pain; (2) Deal with the back problem, but faster and less thoroughly than you usually would; or (3) Refuse and arrange a further appointment. All three have their pros and cons. Option 1 will satisfy the patient but make you run late. Option 2 risks your making a clinical error. Option 3, though defensible, could antagonise the patient and strain the doctor–patient relationship.

Your immediate goal is to make a rapid decision as to which is best, bearing in mind that keeping the patient safe is your primary concern. To do this, you need quickly to establish the presence or absence of red flag symptoms such as a history of trauma, leg weakness or numbness, saddle anaesthesia, bladder or bowel disturbance, fever, or symptoms suggestive of cancer. If any of these are present, only option 1 is open to you, and you will need to go through the full *Patient's part* → *Doctor's part* → *Shared part* sequence. If not (which is more likely), you could go with either option 2 or 3, the decision being affected by such factors as how long it might take to deal with the back pain, what effect over-running might have on your other waiting patients, and the risk of misjudging the problem in your haste.

How you can make it happen

It will be a recurring theme in this section that whenever a patient's behaviour puts you in difficulty, thinking aloud – non-judgementally explaining your dilemma – can be a powerful and effective strategy, and is my personal recommendation. So you could begin by saying something like, 'That puts me in a bit of a spot. I'd like to help, of course, but we've already spent this appointment time on your migraine, and if I now deal with your back, that's going to make me late for my other patients. I'm not sure how urgent it is.' The patient's response will help you make your decision: 'It won't take a moment, I just want some advice,' or 'OK, I'll make another appointment,' or 'Sorry, but I've had to take today off work to see you and I can't afford to keep doing that.'

An alternative would be to use a two-part steer: 'So your back has been painful. Can I just ask you some questions to see whether it's something that needs to be dealt with today?' And then you run through your red-flag questions.

Assuming there is nothing to suggest a clinical emergency, and if you decide nevertheless to offer a shortened secondary consultation about the back pain, I think you are justified in imposing some structure on the Patient's part: 'Tell me how it came on, how it's affecting you, and what you think has caused it.' The Doctor's part, including physical examination, can also be tightly focused, and you can be forgiven if the Shared part is more doctor-centred than usual. Be careful, though, not to let haste or irritation impair your clinical vigilance. Beware of hearing only what you want to hear, finding only what you expect to find, and advising what you always do. In these circumstances, it is especially important to safety net and to offer a follow-up appointment.

If, on the other hand, you are disinclined to deal with the back problem, try to explain why in a non-critical way that the patient can understand and accept. Here again, thinking aloud is a good way of doing this: 'Back pain is not as straightforward a problem as people sometimes think, and it needs time to go into. So now I'm reassured that there are no really urgent features in your case, I'd like to make another time for us to look into it properly. I'm sorry to be difficult, but let's book the appointment now.'

Scenario #2

A 16-year-old girl attends alone, requesting treatment for mild facial acne. She doesn't seem particularly interested in any of your suggestions, but 6 or 7 minutes into the consultation, she suddenly blurts out, 'Can I get the pill from you?'

What needs to happen?

You have the same three options as for the woman with the back pain – *Yes*; *Yes, but quickly*; or *No*. In this case (unless it transpires the youngster means the 'morning after pill'), there is no clinical urgency. But there is a degree of psychological urgency that was absent in the previous scenario. The pill request is clearly the teenager's priority agenda, though it has taken some courage on her part to raise it. The acne was her 'ticket of admission,' and you appear to have passed the Can this doctor be trusted? test. It would be hard-hearted and insensitive, a betrayal even, to turn her away. The immediate question facing you is not whether you will or won't accept the change of topic, but rather how much of a potentially lengthy consultation needs to be undertaken today and how much can safely be deferred to a follow-up appointment.

I expect your usual agenda for a 'going on the pill' consultation, in addition to exploring the background to the patient's request, would include such topics as relationship counselling; menstrual history; the UK medical eligibility criteria; possible alternative methods of contraception; explanation of how to take the pill; side effects and interactions; confidentiality issues; form-filling and data entry; and much else besides. This is a lot to cram into a single full-length consultation, let alone one already abbreviated by the acne discussion. It will not be realistic to attempt to cover all points on this occasion; but if you seem to be trying to cut too many corners, you risk jeopardising what is potentially a very important doctor–patient relationship. Managing this situation calls for you to exercise your professional judgement in prioritising and compromising – two key skills for the general practitioner.

How you can make it happen

An important first step is for you to accept the inevitable: this 'pill consultation within a consultation' needs to follow the entire *Patient's part* → *Doctor's part* → *Shared part* sequence, and is going to over-run. You will be tempted to curtail the Patient's part, but try to resist doing so. You will have more room in the Doctor's and Shared parts to manoeuvre and set limits to what is covered on this occasion.

In response to the girl's 'Can I get the pill?'—you could use the receipt technique: 'That sounds really important, and I guess it's probably the main reason you came today. I'll certainly help. Tell me what you have in mind.' The information you glean in the Patient's part that follows will give you an indication of how much she knows already. It will also help you decide what topics and clinical actions are priorities for today, and what can be deferred. In the Doctor's part, you will want to know details of her menstrual cycle, including the dates of her last and next expected periods, in order to judge how much time you have available (assuming there are no contraindications) before she would need to start her first pill cycle.

When you come to the Shared part, thinking aloud is always a good way to start. Clearly, the details of what you say will reflect the priorities you have inferred from what has gone before. But something like this might be appropriate: 'Yes, I can certainly prescribe the pill for you. It's a big decision, and there are quite a lot of things we need to talk about that we won't have time for today. So ideally, I'd like you to come for another appointment just as soon as we can fix it. And I can give you some written information to read in the meantime. Would that be OK? And is there anything in particular you'd like me to tell you about while you're here today?'

And in your subsequent discussion, you'll draw on some of the general points made earlier in the section on the Shared part: explaining, allowing choice, checking for understanding, safety-netting and so on.

One final point; in *The Inner Consultation* I highlighted the importance of 'housekeeping' – looking after your own stress levels, so that you don't carry the after-effects of one difficult consultation into your dealings with the patients you see afterwards. *'While I'm here'* consultations are inevitably stressful and often result in subsequent patients being kept waiting, and the resulting guilty feeling can make you rushed, flustered or error-prone. If you recognise this possibility, don't be embarrassed to take a few moments to regain your equilibrium. You could, for instance, have a word with your receptionist; she may tell you you've had a lucky cancellation, or perhaps could have a word with the waiting patients and offer apologies for your having been delayed.

The potentially time-consuming consultation

The average GP consultation[4] in Sweden lasts 23 minutes. In the United States, it's 21 minutes[5]; in France, 18 minutes. Of the major European nations, only Germany is below the United Kingdom in the rankings on 8 minutes. Most British GPs are frustrated that the typical 10-minute consultation is not long enough for them to do justice to the number and complexity of the problems their patients present.

EXAM POINT: 10- or 12-minute consultations?

As you know, each SCA case lasts 12 minutes, plus 3 minutes between cases for you to read the notes or background material. In real life, general practice patients are typically booked at 10-minute intervals, so time pressure ought, if anything, to be less during the SCA. On the other hand, there is no possibility of extending an SCA case beyond that 12-minute limit (unless a 'reasonable adjustment' has been previously agreed by the Exam Department). And under exam conditions, when you're trying extra hard to be thorough, the tendency is for consultations to take a little longer.

My personal advice is that by the time you sit the SCA, you should be reasonably comfortable seeing real-life patients booked for 10-minute appointments. If your routine consultations are averaging more than 12 minutes, you may struggle to cover the necessary ground in an SCA case and will probably lose marks, particularly in the 'clinical management and medical complexity' domain.

---

[4] 2017 data.
[5] That's assuming you're not one of the 60,000,000 (approximately) Americans who can't afford to see a family doctor at all.

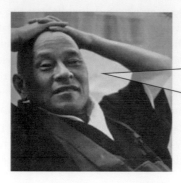

The most important thing is to find out what is the most important thing

Zen master
Shunryu Suzuki
(1904–1971)

FIGURE 5.3

It is worth remembering that the '10-minute appointment' is determined not by legislation or divine ordinance but by arithmetic. If you take the acceptable length of a GP's working day, subtract the time needed for everything other than consulting, and divide by the number of people wanting to be seen, the answer is about 10 minutes. Allocating each patient a specific 10-minute slot is an administrative convenience, not a contract. And if some of those appointments happen to over-run, it isn't a crime or a catastrophe – it's just one of those things. Patients understand this better than the people who design Government targets and patient satisfaction questionnaires. It's only in the SCA exam that every consultation in a booked surgery will run exactly on time (Figure 5.3).[6]

That said, there are circumstances when a consultation's potential agenda is so impracticably long as to threaten major disruption to your timetable. Examples include:

- new diagnosis of a serious or long-term condition;
- an emotional, psychological or family crisis, e.g. bereavement, alcoholism, sexual abuse;
- bad news,[7] e.g. unexpected signs of bony secondaries reported on a routine X-ray.

If the situation confronting you is a clinical emergency, such as an acutely suicidal patient, you have no choice; the consultation will take as long as

---

[6] Note to SCA candidates: this is the only time, too, when each patient should have only one problem, you won't be interrupted, and you won't have to make notes. In fact, you will never have it so good again!

[7] There is a separate section on breaking bad news later in this chapter on 'Some particular challenges.'

it takes. In other circumstances, however, a degree of compromise is possible and necessary. 'Important' is not the same as 'urgent'; some aspects of management, although important, can safely be delegated or postponed. Not everything has to be done on one occasion, or by you. No consultation in general practice needs to be a one-off; there is always the option of a further appointment. Prioritising is the name of the game, and some general principles can be stated:

1   *'Safety first'*: whatever needs to be done to deal with an immediate threat to the patient's life or health must be done immediately.

2   Items of medical management can be triaged into
    - important and time-dependent, i.e. urgent
    - important but not time-dependent, i.e. can, if necessary, be postponed in the short term
    - less important, i.e. probably *should* be delegated or postponed to the medium term

3   Your medical priorities and the patient's personal priorities may not be the same, but they are equally important.

4   Patients need time for any initial strong emotion to subside to a level where they can think and discuss their situation rationally, even if this means delaying some of your agenda.[8]

5   Safety-netting is even more important in consultations where significant medical agenda is deferred.

6   You should make unambiguous notes of what has and has not been covered, and of your follow-up arrangements.

Scenario

A week ago, a 52-year-old man saw the practice nurse for some vaccinations, and mentioned that he had been feeling tired for a few weeks. She found a trace of glycosuria in a urine sample and arranged some blood tests, which have shown a random blood glucose of 12.5 mmol/l and an HbA1c of 55 mmol/mol (7.5%). She telephoned him to say that he probably has diabetes and that he should see the GP. When he enters your room today, he is clearly agitated and blurts out, 'This is terrible, Doctor. My father had diabetes, and he lost his legs to it. And I *must* keep driving.'

---

[8] There is a separate section on dealing with emotional patients in this chapter also.

What needs to happen?

We will probably agree that today's 'must achieve' goals include:

- confirming the provisional diagnosis of type 2 diabetes;
- making or arranging some baseline physical and physiological observations;
- deciding whether and what immediate treatment is appropriate;
- calming the patient's anxieties about the seriousness of his condition, specifically his fear of amputations and driving restrictions;
- establishing a good relationship as a basis for ongoing care.

But the list of other tasks you will want to carry out in the name of good care is very long indeed, certainly far more than could possibly be completed in a single consultation. Here are just some. Under each subheading, I have not made any attempt to prioritise the items; the whole point is that it is for you to make your own judgement in a real-life situation with a real patient.

History: Current symptoms. Complications. Family history. Smoking and alcohol use. Erectile dysfunction. Cardiovascular risk factors. Patient's ideas, concerns and expectations. Employment status. Details of family and social networks.

Examination and investigations: Body mass index. Blood pressure. Lipid profile and other baseline blood tests. Central and peripheral nervous system examination. Peripheral pulses. Visual acuity. Fundoscopy. Examination for skin changes.

Patient information and advice: Diet. Exercise. Smoking and alcohol advice. Long-term sequelae and complications. Foot care. Legal implications for driving. Support groups. Referral to a structured education programme. Flu and Pneumococcus immunisations. Free prescription advice.

Administrative: Practice diabetic register. Setting up computerised recall and monitoring arrangements. QOF protocols.

How you can make it happen

Look through the items on this daunting checklist and triage their urgency into *Action today*, *Soon* or *Later*. Ask yourself what could be delegated. How much can the patient cope with during this appointment, when he is struggling to come to terms with the idea of having a chronic and (he imagines) serious health problem? What is really important for him to understand right from the outset? Of the various items you will postpone till a later occasion, what will you 'signpost' at this stage so that he knows what lies ahead, and what will you leave unmentioned for fear of confusing him with an overload of information?

What consultation strategy will give you the best chance of achieving today's priority goals? The running theme throughout this book is *patient's agenda before doctor's*. Your own clinical agenda of diagnosis and management is not 'life-or-death' urgent; you can afford to let it wait a few minutes until the Doctor's part. The patient is more likely to be receptive to what you have to say if he is first allowed space in the Patient's part for his initial agitation to subside and for his own thoughts and anxieties to be expressed. So you might begin with a receipt: 'You're clearly worried, and that's perfectly understandable. But if you *do* have diabetes, I promise you it's not going to be anything like as bad as you might be imagining. Now – tell me what's led up to you being here today.'

The Doctor's part will consist mainly of you explaining and organising what, in your judgement, is medically necessary at this stage – confirmatory blood tests; whatever baseline investigations and examination you decide to carry out today; and your proposals for his initial treatment. These actions belong in the Doctor's part because they are not really up for discussion; it is your responsibility to make sure they happen. The Shared part will be largely taken up with questions and forward planning, and could be effectively introduced by some thinking aloud: 'That's a lot to take in, and there is much more information I can give you in due course. But most of it we can leave until the next time I see you. What would help me now is to know where your own thoughts are at the moment.'

In short, faced with a consultation that looks liable to over-run – prioritise. Don't bite off more than either of you can comfortably chew. Do today only what needs to be done today; and make sure your plans for completing the agenda are securely in place.

A question of style, values and organisation?

It is difficult for a GP to be both popular and punctual. In our resource-strapped times, patients' legitimate hopes that their doctor will be sympathetic, thorough and unrushed cannot always be met if consultations are routinely booked at 10-minute intervals. If your priority is to keep to time, the only way to do so is to become more doctor-centred and to address only the surface problem while disregarding the depths. If, on the other hand, you prefer to be sympathetic and thorough, you will usually run late. But you can't have it both ways.

The Hollywood screenwriter Robert McKee used to say that 'a character's values are revealed by the choices they make under pressure.' When the building is on fire, do you save the girl or the diamonds? Your response to finding yourself under time pressure reflects your professional values as much as the practical realities. There may, of course, be perfectly valid reasons for needing your surgeries to run punctually: child care and other domestic or social commitments, for example. But the challenge posed by time-needy patients forces you to confront your ideas of what good practice consists of and what sort of doctor you want to be.

While good consulting skills will help you strike the best balance between effectiveness and efficiency, they can never be a complete answer to time pressure. Constantly feeling you don't have enough time for patients is often the result of organisational and administrative factors that arise, and must be dealt with, outside the consulting room. Does the practice, for example, consistently under-estimate the number of appointments needed? Are there enough doctors working enough sessions? Is there enough flexibility in the availability of doctors and the appointment system? Is there the right mix of face-to-face and remote (telephone or video) consultations? Are the receptionists sufficiently trained in triaging patients' requests to be seen? Is the best use being made of colleagues such as practice nurses, nurse practitioners, physician assistants, pharmacists and counsellors? Is the practice's policy on using locums overly parsimonious?

Long-agenda consultations in the SCA

An anxiety commonly expressed by candidates preparing for the SCA by practising mock cases – the scenario described above could well be one – is, 'There simply isn't enough time to cover everything.' Exactly; that is the point. 'Everything' is not what you should attempt to cover. Trying to do so rather suggests that you are still thinking like a doctor in hospital practice, where every 'i' must be dotted and every 't' crossed. In the SCA, trying to cram 20-minutes-worth of agenda into 12 minutes will probably go against you, because it shows a lack of empathy for a patient who can't be expected to take it all in. The examiners, who are all practising GPs themselves, will be very happy if they see that you can prioritise and do what needs to be done today and make appropriate follow-up plans for whatever there isn't time for.

The uncommunicative patient

Scenario

You: 'How can I help?'
Patient: 'It's my back.'
You: 'Your back?

Patient: 'Yes.'
You: 'What about your back?'
Patient: 'It hurts.'
You: 'Tell me more about it.'
Patient: 'What do you want to know?'

At this point, you could be forgiven for thinking, *This is like trying to get blood out of a stone*, giving up on the Patient's part as a lost cause, and moving straight on to the Doctor's part, probably with a series of closed questions:

You: 'How long has it been painful?'
Patient: 'A fair while.'
You: 'A few days? Weeks? Months?'
Patient: 'Weeks, maybe.'
You: 'Does the pain go down your legs?'
Patient: 'Not really.'

Even if you try to stay in the Patient's part by asking open questions about, for example, ideas, concerns and expectations, you may be met with equally frustrating answers:

You: 'What did you think might be causing it?'
Patient: 'I don't know, you're the doctor.'
You: 'Was there anything you were worried it might be?'
Patient: *(Shrugs)*
You: 'How would you like me to help?'
Patient: 'Well, I need it sorted.'

Thankfully, few patients are quite as exasperating as this. But some patients are undoubtedly difficult to get into 'telling-the-doctor-all-about-it' mode. This is not because they are trying to be awkward. If they are elderly, it is probable that they have had long experience of doctor-led consultations being the norm. There may be cultural or socioeconomic reasons, too, for being what we might regard as excessively deferential to doctors.

What needs to happen?

The uncommunicative patient is just as likely to have important psychological, emotional and social components to his problem as others who find it easy to pour their hearts out. It would be just as helpful to know his thoughts and priorities, even though they might be hard to extract.

Nevertheless, it is very easy, faced with such tight-lipped reticence, to abandon the Patient's part as a lost cause. But it is important to resist the temptation to switch to a heavily doctor-centred style of data-gathering, and to do your best to encourage the patient out of his initial passivity and into 'telling-the-doctor-all-about-it' mode if at all possible. If this proves too hard, you may still be able to preserve the important distinction between Patient's and Doctor's parts by the nature of the questions you pose.

Thinking ahead to the Shared part, where the patient's participation is particularly valuable, it would be good in the early stages of the consultation to have the patient see the benefits of being actively involved in the discussion.

How you can make it happen

Process awareness is important, i.e. recognising what is going on in time to do something about it. The impatient feeling you get in this situation is a warning that you are in danger: in danger of over-reacting through frustration and taking premature control of the consultation instead of persevering with the collaborative approach you know is ultimately to be preferred. Your first goal is not to yield to this temptation but to try to create a meaningful Patient's part.

As to tactics, it is worth sticking with open questions. Don't give up at the first hurdle.

You: 'Tell me more about it.'
Patient: 'What do you want to know?'
You: 'I'd like to know as much as possible about the problem, from your point of view. Could you tell me about it, from the start?'

You could also try 'semi-open questions' – questions that suggest some paragraph headings for the story you would like the patient to tell you, without being too specific or restrictive.

You: 'Tell me more about it.
Patient: 'What do you want to know?'
You: 'I'd like to know how it all started, and how it's affecting you.'

In the Patient's part, semi-open questions can offer a tongue-tied patient just enough structure to kick-start their own account. Here are some more examples that might be effective in eliciting particular aspects of the patient's story:

- 'What happened next?' (clarifying the sequence of events)
- 'What went through your mind at that point? (ideas or concerns)

- 'How did it make you feel?' (psychological impact)
- 'What's going on in your life at the moment?' (social context)
- 'What was it that made you decide to come and see me?' (priorities, health beliefs)
- 'What do you know about possible treatments?' (expectations)

Even if you *do* find yourself asking a string of closed questions that should really belong in the Doctor's part, it is worth slipping in an occasional open question in case the patient is now able to be a bit more forthcoming:

You: 'Is it worse in the morning or the evening?'
Patient: 'It gets worse as the day goes on.'
You: 'Any change in your bowels or waterworks?'
Patient: 'No.'
You: 'So what would you say has been the most worrying thing about it?'
Patient: 'I suppose, if it doesn't improve, I might have to start looking for another job.'

When the patient begins to volunteer some unprompted information, it's a good idea to give a receipt and some words of encouragement:

Patient: 'I mean, everyone gets backache, don't they? I just thought it would go if I rested it.'
You: 'You're right, it often does. But in your case, it sounds as if it's got worse.'

One useful linguistic trick is to ask, 'Would you be willing to start be telling me as much as you can about what's been happening?' There is something about being asked, 'Would you be willing …?' that evokes the answer, 'Yes, certainly.'

Another strategy (as always, when you are in difficulty) is to think aloud. For example:

> The more you can tell me about the problem in your own words, the easier it is for me to understand how it's affecting you.

or

> The way I like to work is, first, I'd like you to tell me as much as you can about your problem in your own words, and then there are some questions I'll want to ask you about it.

Another point when you will want to encourage a reticent patient's contribution comes as you begin the Shared part. Some clear signposting is helpful:

> OK, we'll move on now and discuss how to get you better. I'll start by telling you what I think is going on, and what the possible treatments are, and then I'd like you to tell me what you think about what I say.

Uncommunicative role-players in the SCA

There is a belief amongst some SCA candidates that the role-play patients have been instructed to be difficult and to deliberately play 'hard to get.' This is untrue; they have not. On the other hand, this being an exam and one-third of the marks being for data gathering, it is unlikely that a simple 'Tell me all about it' will be enough to unleash the disclosure of all relevant information. The only scripted part of the role-player's brief is the opening words; what happens after that is governed, as it is in real life, largely by your own approach. Again, as in real life, the role-play patient will find it easier to open up to you if you establish a good rapport and appear interested and helpful. So you should begin each SCA consultation as you would any other, by being friendly, sounding interested, paying good attention, starting with open questions, and developing the Patient's part in the ways we have been considering.

EXAM POINT: Role-players v. Real patients

Candidates sometimes fear that role-played consultations won't show them in their best light, as knowing that the 'patient' isn't real distorts their performance. However, in practice, any sense of artificiality quickly subsides, and there is no evidence that a doctor's behaviour in a role-played consultation is significantly different from their usual consulting style. Simulated patients are extensively used at every stage of medical education, so you will almost certainly be familiar with them already. The role players in the SCA are highly trained professional actors, and their performance and consistency are closely monitored for quality assurance.

In some ways, consultations in the SCA are easier than in real life. As a rule, the 'patient' will have only one problem, and it will be a problem that can be adequately managed in 12 minutes. And they won't be irritatingly talkative or frustratingly monosyllabic. As part of preparing for the exam, get plenty of practice with role-played consultations, using your colleagues and peers to play the patient role.

The over-talkative patient

Scenario

The patient is a 50-year-old woman, widowed two years ago, who works in a school canteen. As soon as she sits down, she begins, 'I hope I'm not wasting your time, Doctor, because I know how busy you are, and I wouldn't ordinarily come. I can't remember the last time, not since Derek passed away, God rest his soul, I do miss him. It's just I was telling my friend Jean – we go to this line dancing class, don't laugh, because I do try to keep my weight down, honestly, not that you'll believe me. Anyway, she said I ought to come because, well, I just feel so tired all the time. It's like I've got no energy at all, and that's not like me, normally there aren't enough hours in the day. And it's not as if I'm not sleeping; as soon as my head hits the pillow, I'm off. I did wonder if I might be anaemic, because they do say, don't they, iron and what-not. But I eat pretty well; I mean, look at the size of me. But we're all big-boned in my family, and I'm not vegan or anything, so I should be getting all my vitamins …'

Sometimes you feel like throttling those so-called consultation experts who tell you to begin by encouraging the patient to tell you the problem in their own words.

What needs to happen?

People with such strong pressure to keep talking often do so for fear of finding a well of emptiness inside themselves if they stop. Nevertheless, unless you do something to control and focus the relentless stream of words, you will get cross and risk making an error of judgement, and the consultation is in danger of over-running. Amongst the irrelevancies are several cues to what might be important factors in the patient's complaint. But it can be difficult to detect these signals against the high level of background noise, or to act on them, without interrupting the patient.

Interrupt you *must*. Good patient-centred practice requires you to ensure the time available is used to maximum effectiveness, and that cannot be done unless you can prune the rambling narrative as you would a rose, so that it can ultimately bloom to full advantage. But it needs to be done as kindly as possible, without hurting the patient's feelings.

How you can make it happen

As with the previous uncommunicative patient, your feeling of mounting irritation is the signal that you need to take active steps to keep the consultation on a productive track. The longer you let the monologue continue, the harder it will be to break the pattern.

One way of doing this is to rein back on some of your normal rapport-building narrative-encouraging behaviour. You could reduce your eye contact a bit; be less generous with your 'Uh-huh's and 'Mmm's; perhaps ease your chair fractionally away from the patient's. Slightly stronger would be for you to raise a hand, palm toward the patient, in the gesture that means 'Whoa!' and say, 'Could I just stop you there for a moment?' Then give a two-part steer: 'You've mentioned a few things that might have a bearing on your tiredness. Could you tell me more about ...'

'Tell me more about' *what*? Embedded within the patient's saga are pointers to several possible reasons for her tiredness: depression following bereavement; increasing bodyweight; anaemia. In the absence of anything more definite, you would have to follow your nose, suggest a topic for her to elaborate on, and see where it leads.

Another strategy is to interject frequent mini-summaries: 'You're still grieving for your husband'; 'It sounds like you're very conscious of your weight'; 'So you'd considered anaemia as a possible reason.' When you think you have gleaned as much as you are going to from the Patient's part, a firmly-turned receipt will help you move into the Doctor's part: 'Thank you. What you've told me is very helpful. But we only have limited time today, so now I'm going to ask you some specific medical questions.'

The challenge to your communication skills is how to impose the necessary degree of control without appearing discourteous or unsympathetic. Can you think of some more polite ways of saying, 'Anyway, to cut a long story short ...?'

The emotional patient

We know from neuroscience that the part of the brain that mediates emotion, the limbic system, is, in evolutionary terms, longer established than the cerebral cortex, and its activity cannot be completely overridden by rational thought. Emotion is also a partly biochemical process, subject to the effects of adrenaline and other neurotransmitters, all of which, once in play, take a finite time to dissipate. You can't quickly talk away an emotion, and you can't think straight while in the grip of one. Telling someone in a violent rage to calm down actually makes it worse, and you wouldn't dream of asking someone in floods of tears if they could weep a little faster.

There is an emotional component in virtually every consultation, not always affecting solely the patient. In most cases, this is not intense enough to affect how the consultation plays out. But sometimes it is, so it is as well to have some general principles for handling emotions when they arise.

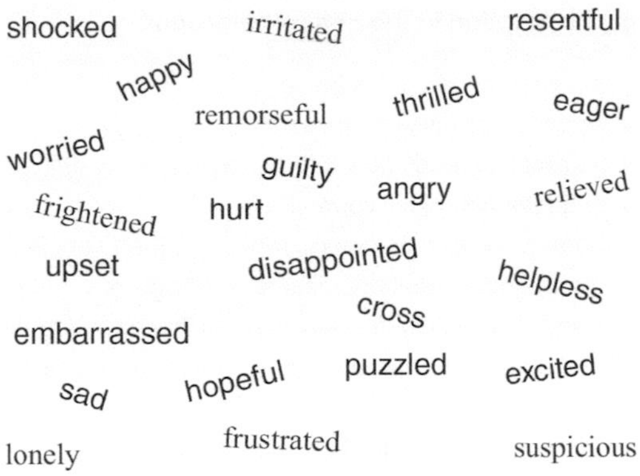

shocked   irritated   resentful

happy

worried   remorseful   thrilled   eager

guilty   angry   relieved

frightened   hurt

upset   disappointed   helpless

cross

embarrassed

sad   hopeful   puzzled   excited

lonely   frustrated   suspicious

FIGURE 5.4

Displays of extreme emotion are rare in general practice but have a powerful impact when they do occur: the despairing grief of the unexpectedly bereaved; the accusing fury of someone who holds you responsible for some tragedy; the frantic dread of a newly diagnosed sufferer from motor neurone disease as an imagined future begins to dawn. Much more common are shifting undercurrents of emotion causing ripples on the surface of the consultation that every now and then become too strong to ignore.

Figure 5.4 shows a selection of words describing feelings that may emerge and become evident in the course of a consultation. Have you encountered any patients for whom this has happened? Can you imagine circumstances when they might? Have you yourself ever had such feelings in the course of your work? Or in your personal life? Can you think of any others not included in the box?

When strong emotions arise, addressing them needs to become your immediate priority. It is pointless to try and carry on as if it wasn't happening. If you don't deal with it, or at least acknowledge it and allow it to be expressed, it will distort and frustrate the rest of the consultation. Insofar as it is possible to generalise, I suggest the following strategy (see Figure 5.5).

1 **Recognise what the patient is feeling,** from what they say or how they look or behave. Your own life experience as a human being helps you to empathise, i.e. to imagine how another person is probably feeling.

2 **Acknowledge and name the patient's emotion.** It is reassuring to have one's feelings validated and given a name. You may well have a better emotional vocabulary than the patient; choosing the right word demonstrates your empathy and shows the patient that what they are feeling is something well-known and understandable. Don't just say,

Dealing with emotion in the consulting room

- Recognise what the patient is feeling
- Acknowledge it, and give it a name
- Accept the emotion, and allow it to be expressed (within reason)
- Try not to react emotionally yourself
- Expect the emotion to crescendo, peak, and then subside
- After the emotion has peaked, discuss it rationally
- Make a plan, if necessary, for dealing with its consequences
- Resume the consultation where you left off, or from wherever the emotion has left you
- Remember you may need to do some 'housekeeping'

FIGURE 5.5

'I know how you're feeling.' Better would be 'You're looking sad', or 'You sound quite worried', or 'I think you find that rather frightening', or 'In your situation I think I'd be pretty annoyed.'

Match the strength of the emotion with the strength of the word describing it; someone who is clearly furious will not accept being told they are 'a bit miffed.'

3 **Accept the emotion as it is,** and, within socially acceptable limits, allow the patient to express it. Help the patient put their feelings into words. Show your acceptance by active listening or non-verbally, e.g. through touch or by offering a tissue. If the patient is angry, allow a verbal rant, but make it clear that personal abuse, threats or intimidation are not acceptable.

4 **Don't react emotionally yourself,** if possible You haven't caused the patient's emotion, and it isn't about you personally. Try not to get defensive or critical or argumentative.

5 **Most emotions crescendo, reach a maximum, then begin to subside.** When you sense that peak intensity has passed, you can begin to suggest discussing it. A two-part steer is useful here, e.g. 'I understand how angry this has made you. Is it something we could talk about?' or, 'I'm glad you were able to cry. Where are your thoughts now?'

6 **Discuss the situation rationally.** Once the emotion has subsided to manageable levels, discuss what led to it and what its implications are for the future. Don't be surprised if there are 'aftershocks' at this point, i.e. secondary, less intense shows of the previous emotion.

7 **Make a considered plan,** if necessary, for dealing with any issues that have arisen.

8 **Resume the consultation.** Pick up where you left off; or, if the emotion has changed the agenda, begin a new 'consultation within a consultation.'

9 **Monitor and manage your own emotional state.** If find your own emotions have been triggered, you may need to do some 'housekeeping,' i.e. taking care of yourself after the consultation has ended. You might, for instance, need a cup of tea, or a chat with a colleague, or a brief spell out of the consulting room.

This final point, dealing with your own emotions, is important. Emotion in a patient inevitably induces some degree of emotional response in you, the doctor. This may be an empathic 'resonance,' where, to some extent, you share the patient's feelings. Sometimes, however, the patient's emotion may involve you or be directed towards you, in which case you may experience some reactive countertransference; for instance, feelings of resentment if the patient is inappropriately blaming you for something. Either way, it is common to feel a rush of adrenaline when a patient becomes emotionally aroused, resulting in the primitive 'fight or flight' response. If you feel this is starting to happen, try to maintain process awareness. Try to dissociate from your instinctive reaction and observe what is going on in the interaction between you and the patient. Asking yourself, *What am I feeling and why?* can sometimes lead to interesting insights into the patient's own problem.[9]

Scenario

The patient is a 35-year-old man who seldom attends the surgery, although you are the usual doctor for his wife and two young children. He looks rather shamefaced and says, 'I've got a problem, Doctor. A gambling problem. I suppose you'd say I'm an addict, and I've got to do something about it.' Already you feel a plan forming in your mind: screen for depression, suggest Gamblers Anonymous or Citizens Advice ... Abruptly he breaks off, puts his head in his hands and begins to weep inconsolably. In between sobs, the story emerges: it's been going on for years; he's massively in debt; his wife had no idea until she saw his credit card statement last week. 'She's left me, and taken the kids. I can't blame her. And now it's looks like we'll lose the house. It's the end of the road for me.' And his weeping resumes even more intensely.

What needs to happen?

A good outcome for this consultation would be if you could establish a working relationship – a 'therapeutic alliance' – with the patient, move

---

[9] This approach of noticing and reflecting on one's own emotional responses lies at the heart of the Balint tradition which has contributed so much to the study of the consultation process. For a fuller study of this phenomenon, see my book *The Inner Physician*.

him from his present negativity towards a more optimistic outlook, and begin to formulate a recovery plan.

How you can make it happen

While he is still in the throes of desperation, the patient will not be accessible to any discussion of a plan of action. You need to deal with his emotional state first.

What is he feeling? Ashamed? Guilty? Self-pitying? Self-loathing? Scared? Remorseful? Probably all of these. What can you say that will show you understand? Possibly something like this:

You: 'It sounds like things seem pretty hopeless at the moment.'
Patient: 'Mmmm.' *(He weeps some more.)*
You: 'And maybe a bit ashamed? Guilty, maybe? Scared?'
Patient: 'All of that.'

If he now looks up and makes eye contact with you, he is probably starting to feel the sense of connection that comes from being understood. Perhaps he is ready to talk more about his situation. And perhaps if you use his first name, it will help him to confide in you.

You: 'Jeremy – it *is* Jeremy, isn't it …?'
Patient: 'My friends call me Jez. Except I don't have any friends left.'

And he lapses back into weeping; his emotion has not yet sufficiently run its course to allow calm discussion. If you keep a box of tissues handy for situations like this, you could offer it, but not too soon, lest it be seen as a signal that you think it's time to stop crying now. Before long, Jeremy (being British and male) 'pulls himself together,' says, 'Sorry about that,' and begins to tell you the chain of events leading to his coming to see you. He is now into the Patient's part, and the rest of the consultation can follow the usual *Patient's part → Doctor's part → Shared part* sequence, bearing in mind that it may be interrupted from time to time if his emotions well up again. The Doctor's part will include assessing his mental health and suicide risk, and in the Shared part, you can suggest involving other agencies as well as offering (I hope) your own personal support as well.

Breaking bad news

It is not often that a general practice consultation is the locus for a truly devastating information bombshell, compared, say, with an Accident and Emergency department or Oncology outpatients. On a daily basis, our hospital colleagues in these settings have to break the news of catastrophic disruption to the life of a hitherto unsuspecting patient. Nevertheless, there are occasions when we GPs have to tell a patient something that means they will probably leave the consulting room feeling more worried than when they came in. Unexpectedly abnormal test results; confirmation of a life-changing disease; disclosing and explaining the contents of a consultant's letter; situations like these represent a reversal of the usual order, where it is the patient who brings a problem for the doctor's attention. Here, the GP must present the patient with an unexpected or unwelcome problem – and then pick up the pieces.

The two parts of that last sentence – give the patient the problem and then pick up the pieces – provide a clue to how a 'breaking bad news' consultation can best be handled: in two parts.

Think of it as two consecutive 'consultations within a consultation,' each with its own *Patient's part → Doctor's part → Shared part* structure. (I'll use the acronym CWAC for a Consultation Within A Consultation.) Overall, the consultation consists of CWAC #1 followed by CWAC #2. CWAC #1 comprises the doctor telling the patient what the news is and making sure that the facts are understood. CWAC #2 is dealing with the impact on the patient of the news, and planning what to do about it. Figure 5.6 illustrates this.

The first 'consultation within a consultation' – giving the news

If you know this is going to be a 'bad news' consultation, take a few moments before the patient's arrival to marshal your information and your thoughts. Make sure you have read the notes, the pathology results or the relevant correspondence. Run over in your mind the key points you will want to communicate, and think how you are going to express them sensitively but unambiguously.

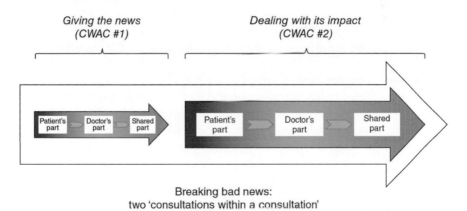

Breaking bad news:
two 'consultations within a consultation'

FIGURE 5.6

The Patient's part of CWAC #1 – the patient's version of the reason for coming – is often quite brief. It might be:

'I've come for the results of my X-ray,' or
'The nurse did a heart tracing, and she said something about an irregular heartbeat,' or
'I gather you've had a letter from the hospital.'

Whether in an attempt to 'soften the blow' or to put off the painful moment, it can be tempting to prolong the Doctor's part of CWAC #1 by recapping at length the history of the patient's problem, or dwelling too long on the ideas, concerns and expectations agenda. But keeping the patient on tenterhooks like this is *not* an act of kindness:

Patient: 'I've come for the results of my X-ray.'
You: 'Yes, I've got it here. Now let me see, you saw my partner last week about a cough you've been having, and she listened to your chest and apparently it sounded OK, but just to be on the safe side she thought it would be wise to get an X-ray. And I agree, because your cough had gone on for some weeks, is that right? Tell me, do you smoke?'
Patient: 'What does the X-ray show?'

Neither is this:

You: 'Before I tell about the X-ray, could you say what you were hoping it would show, what you thought it might possibly be, and whether there is anything you were particularly worried about.'

I think the best strategy is to begin with a short 'warning shot' – a remark that suggests bad news is coming – and then follow quickly with the key points of the information you have to deliver, in lay language, without euphemisms, and if possible, with a note of optimism. For example:

Patient: 'I've come for the results of my X-ray.'
You: 'Yes, I've got the report here. And I'm afraid it shows an abnormal shadow on your right lung, which might just be a bit of infection but unfortunately looks very much like a tumour – a cancer – on the lung. We'll need to get this looked into as quickly as possible.'

Another example:

Patient: 'The nurse did a heart tracing, and she said something about an irregular heartbeat.'

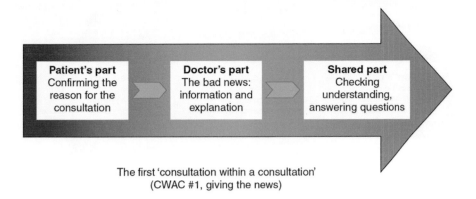

The first 'consultation within a consultation'
(CWAC #1, giving the news)

FIGURE 5.7

You: 'Yes, it's good that she spotted it. The ECG tracing shows you have a condition called atrial fibrillation, which makes your heart beat erratically. It's not too serious in itself, but it could cause complications if we don't take precautions to prevent them.'

Although well-intentioned, euphemisms and circumlocutions such as 'the blood tests weren't exactly normal,' or 'the possibility of something untoward' can raise false hopes and leave room for misunderstanding; in my opinion, they are best avoided.

The Doctor's part in CWAC #1 need be no more than this: a short statement of the facts, together with any explanation necessary. The Shared part of CWAC #1 is similarly brief: making sure the patient understands what has been said so far (see Figure 5.7).

The second 'consultation within a consultation' – dealing with the impact of the news

The news imparted in CWAC #1 transforms the rest of the consultation. The patient must rapidly absorb and process what the doctor has said. Thereafter, an entirely new agenda is generated that had not existed when the patient entered the room a few minutes earlier. The bad news takes the patient to a new place and creates a new problem, which now forms the Patient's part of the second 'consultation within the consultation' (see Figure 5.8). To relate this to the two examples I have used already: in the patient with the abnormal chest X-ray, the news of probable cancer transforms his mildly anxious curiosity into an emotional morass of panic and dread, which is now the focus for the second phase of the consultation. The initial 'The nurse said something

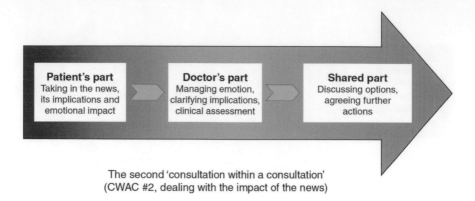

The second 'consultation within a consultation'
(CWAC #2, dealing with the impact of the news)

FIGURE 5.8

about an irregular heartbeat' of the patient with atrial fibrillation becomes an urgent need in CWAC #2, for answers to Helman's six questions.[10]

From this revised starting position, and after allowing 'processing time' for the patient to take in and react to the news, the rest of the consultation can now follow its usual three-part sequence. If, as may well be the case, the patient is emotionally affected by the bad news, this will need to be sympathetically handled in the way described a few pages ago before you move on to the more clinical aspects of the case and its management. In the Doctor's part, you will want to ascertain what support the patient has in facing their new circumstances. In the Shared part, I expect you will reassure the patient of the ongoing support of yourself and your team, and perhaps, once the consultation is over, offer the human comfort of some privacy to regain composure, a cup of tea or the chance to make a phone call to a family member or friend.

The following composite diagram (Figure 5.9) shows how two consecutive 'consultations within a consultation' form a template for most 'bad news' scenarios – and also for consultations where, on the face of it, the news is good.

'Good' news can be bad

Sometimes the information you have to give a patient is that test results are normal, that there is no evidence of disease. You would think, wouldn't you, that this would be good news to be greeted with relief. But not if the patient's problem has a psychosomatic origin, with the patient wanting a physical explanation for symptoms having a psychological or emotional basis. In this

---

[10] Remember Cecil Helman: six questions patients want answered are: What has happened?; Why has it happened?; Why to me?; Why now?; What could happen?; What should be done?

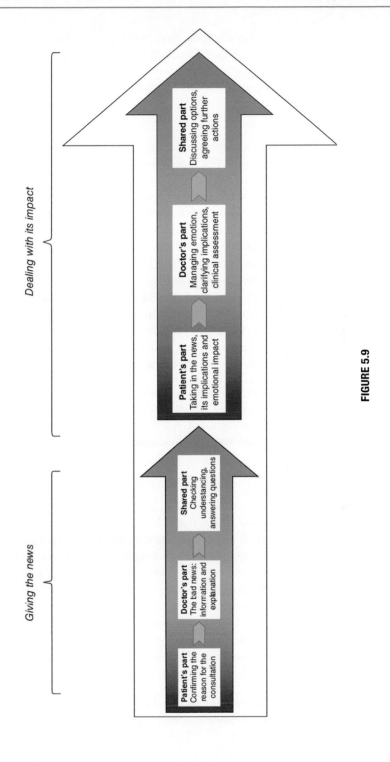

FIGURE 5.9

Giving the news

Patient's part
Confirming the reason for the consultation

Doctor's part
The bad news: information and explanation

Shared part
Checking understanding, answering questions

Dealing with its impact

Patient's part
Taking in the news, its implications and emotional impact

Doctor's part
Managing emotion, clarifying implications, clinical assessment

Shared part
Discussing options, agreeing further actions

situation, news that is clinically good from the doctor's point of view is, to the patient, bad, in that it obliges them to face the uncomfortable possibility that non-physical causes will have to be considered, explored and confronted. The same 'two consultations within a consultation' approach can be effective.

Scenario

The patient is a 27-year-old mother of three who attends frequently with minor illnesses and anxiety. You know from previous consultations that she feels trapped in a loveless and abusive marriage; she would like to leave, taking the children with her, but doesn't know where she would go or how she would support herself. Two weeks ago, she consulted you, complaining of feeling tired all the time, saying, 'I'm sure there's something wrong, my blood or my hormones or something. I shouldn't be this tired.' You asked a range of 'red flag' questions and examined her, finding nothing abnormal, and arranged screening blood tests, including a full blood count, ESR, C-reactive protein, liver and thyroid function tests, fasting blood glucose and serum vitamin D. All results are within their normal ranges. You strongly suspect her tiredness is providing her with a reason for putting off the difficult decision as to whether or not to leave her husband. Today, she attends the planned follow-up appointment.

Patient: 'I hope the tests show why it is I'm so tired.'
You: 'I'm pleased to say they are all normal, no sign of anything wrong anywhere. So that's good, isn't it?'
Patient: 'Really? That can't be right, they must have missed something.'
You: 'No, if there was anything physically the matter it would have shown up.'

With that short exchange, CWAC #1 is complete, leaving the agenda for the rest of the consultation substantially altered. The patient was expecting to be given a diagnosis that would have justified her indecision, but instead, the unconscious defence mechanisms underlying her symptoms will reassert themselves all the more strongly. It is likely that, in the Patient's part of CWAC #2, she will insist she must be suffering from something rare or unusual, that she needs more tests, that perhaps she should see a specialist.

In the Doctor's part of CWAC #2, you will probably want to double-check that you haven't missed any pointers to organic disease. Then, reluctant to over-investigate or make an inappropriate referral, you might try and see how amenable the patient is to considering a psychological explanation.

You: 'I know you're very unhappy at home. I remember you told me once that for two pins you would take the children and leave; and

I was wondering, if you weren't so tired, do you think you might find those two pins and do just that, walk out?[11]'

Patient: 'Probably. I know I can't go on like this, I've got to do something.'

Thinking aloud during the final Shared part, you will probably explain why you consider doing more tests would be a distraction, and that you would prefer her to think things over and come back next week to tell you what she has decided to do.

'Breaking bad news' in the SCA

Breaking bad news can make a good case for the SCA. A typical scenario might be that another clinician has organised some tests or written a letter indicating a serious diagnosis or poor prognosis, and the patient is consulting you in order to be given the information. The challenge should be obvious, provided you have read the case notes in advance.

Before the consultation begins, try to imagine how you would feel if *you* were in the patient's shoes, and what you would want to know. This will help you to avoid a mistake made by some candidates who, through a misunderstanding of what 'patient-centred' means, begin by encouraging the patient into a lengthy re-telling of the history that prompted the tests in the first place, followed by a mostly irrelevant exploration of the ideas, concerns and expectations agenda. This sort of thing:

Patient: 'I think you've got the results of the blood tests your colleague arranged.'

Poor candidate: 'Yes, I have. What was the problem you were having that led to them being done?'

Patient: 'I've been losing weight.'

Poor candidate: 'Tell me more about that. How much weight have you lost? Over what period of time? Do you get breathless?' *(etcetera)*

Patient: 'Isn't that all in the notes?'

Poor candidate: 'Actually, yes. What do you think the tests might show? Is there anything you're worried it could be? And how would you like me to help you today?'

Patient: (thinking but not saying) *I'd like you to help by telling me the* ***** *test results!*

---

[11] When looking for the cause of psychosomatic symptoms, don't spend too much time going into details of the symptoms. It can be more productive to look for the 'secondary gain' – the effect the symptoms are having on the patient's life – and consider the possibility that they are achieving an outcome that the patient desires but is unable or unwilling to express consciously, in this case providing an excuse for avoiding the difficult 'Shall I stay or leave?' decision.

This frustrating inquisition wastes time and antagonises the patient. Better would be the 'two-CWAC' approach, beginning:

Patient:	'I think you've got the results of the blood tests your colleague arranged.'
You:	'These are the tests you had because you'd been losing weight? Yes, they're back, and they show you have an overactive thyroid gland. We'll need to do some more tests to find out why, but ultimately it should be something we can treat quite easily.'

And now you are into the second mini-consultation, beginning with the patient's reaction to the news and leaving you plenty of time to impress the examiner with your skill at explaining and managing hyperthyroidism.

Non-clinical scenarios in the SCA

One new feature of the SCA is that not all 12 cases will consist of consultations with a role-played patient. Real-life general practice often requires a GP to talk to a third party *about* a patient, not directly *to* the patient. To replicate this, at least one scenario will require you to have a discussion with another professional or member of the extended health care team, such as a District Nurse community pharmacist, physiotherapist, social worker or counsellor. Examples (not taken from the actual SCA case bank!) might be: a telephone call from a local pharmacist about a customer asking for stronger analgesic tablets; a conversation with a Macmillan nurse about a young woman recently bereaved; or a request from a police officer for information about a patient of yours who has been arrested for possession of Class A drugs. Scenarios like these may not, at first sight, seem to fit into the *Patient's part–Doctor's part–Shared part* structure described in this book.

However, the principles of the three-part approach still apply and can form the basis for how you handle the situation (see Figure 5.10). First – the equivalent of the *Patient's part* – you begin by encouraging the other person to tell you as much as possible about the issue or problem as it appears to them, including their own ideas about what is going on, their particular concerns, and how they are hoping you will help. Secondly – as in the *Doctor's part* – you need to make sure you have all the factual information necessary for you to make a proper professional assessment of the problem. Finally, by sharing your own thoughts and point of view and following a frank discussion, you should agree a course of action that best meets the priorities of all concerned, concluding with a recap of what has been decided. This approach maps nicely onto the three domains in which every SCA case is marked: data-gathering and diagnosis, clinical management and medical complexity, and relating to others.

Structuring a non-clinical scenario in the SCA

Patient's part: get the story	Doctor's part: do the medicine	Shared part: discuss the plan
Get as full an understanding as you can of the situation as it appears to the other person, including their ideas, concerns & expectations.	Then make sure you have all the factual information you need in order to make a professional assessment. Summarise to confirm your understanding of the issue.	Finally, by discussion and exchange of ideas, agree a course of action that best meets the expectations of all concerned. Recap and document the outcome and the actions that have been agreed.

FIGURE 5.10

Many of the communication skills described in this book will help you to achieve this: active attentive listening; open questions; picking up cues; giving receipts; two-part steers; summarising; and thinking aloud. In addition, non-clinical scenarios will often present you with significant ethical dilemmas or require you to demonstrate your grasp of what is appropriate professional behaviour. There may, for instance, be issues of confidentiality, or informed consent, or safeguarding of children or vulnerable adults. To prepare yourself for these challenges, it is worth familiarising yourself with *Good Medical Practice*, published by the General Medical Council and downloadable from their website.

As an example, suppose you take a telephone call from the head teacher of a local primary school, who tells you that she is worried about a 7-year-old pupil who, together with his family, is a patient of your practice. According to the teacher, the child has recently become tearful and withdrawn. Today in class, he had a nosebleed. It had soon stopped, but his mother was contacted, and she collected him and took him home. However, the teacher had noticed some recent bruising on his arms, which the boy said was the result of a tussle with one of his siblings. She says, 'I just thought I should let you know.'

As with any consultation, you will want to start with open questions and prompts such as, 'Tell me more about it,' 'Do you have any relevant background information?' and 'Is there anything else you think it would be helpful for me to know?' Mirroring the Ideas, Concerns and Expectations agenda of a clinical consultation, you will ask the teacher for her own thoughts about what was going on, what fears or suspicions she had, whether she had taken any steps already, and how she thought you might help in this situation. Moving on to the equivalent of the Doctor's part, you will want to find out if there is any possibility that the child might be at risk, psychologically or physically. What existing policies does the school have for dealing with situations like this? If you don't know the family already, the teacher may be able to tell you whether there is, for instance, any history or suggestion of violence or abuse in the home. You will also probably want to access the medical records of the child and other family members.

The case raises a number of ethical and professional issues, including confidentiality, safeguarding and multidisciplinary working. In considering what to do, you will make the safety and well-being of the child your first priority. You will need to know, or find out, what are the local child protection arrangements if you feel the child is at sufficient risk to justify actioning them, bearing in mind that doing so clumsily or unnecessarily may do serious damage to the family. However, you will be on your guard against jumping to premature conclusions, remembering that there could be a medical reason for the nosebleed and bruising, such as leukaemia. You will probably decide that you need to see the child and parents as soon as possible, and will perhaps discuss with the teacher the best and least alarming way of arranging this. One way might be to contact the child's mother and ask her to bring the child to see you to follow-up the nosebleed. Such a consultation would give you an opportunity to assess the possibility of non-accidental injury or mental health issues.

No doubt you can think of other factors and possible actions that will affect how you would handle the teacher's call. As so often in general practice, there is no single 'right' way of dealing with this complex situation. If this were an SCA case, the examiners would give you credit for arriving at whatever plan will keep the child safe and fulfil your own professional responsibilities, while at the same time reassuring the teacher that both you and she are collaborating in the child's interests.

When it all goes wrong

Your mind goes blank. You forget what you were going to say. With a sinking feeling, you realise you have completely missed the point of the consultation. You and the patient are at cross purposes; the patient is getting annoyed and you are becoming frustrated or embarrassed. You have no idea what to do next, and it's obvious to both of you that you don't know what you're talking about.

We have all had cringe-worthy moments like these. The even worse nightmare is that it's while you're doing the SCA that your brain turns to mush and you imagine the examiner wincing as 9 marks fly out of the window.

Don't panic. This is what you do.

Stop digging: When in a hole, stop digging. Stop. Pause. Carrying on regardless, trying to bluster your way out, will only make things worse.

Own up: Admit that you are in difficulty. Say, 'I'm sorry, my mind's gone a blank.' Or, 'We seem to have got off on the wrong foot.' Or, 'This isn't going well, is it?'

Pause for process awareness: Mentally step back and see if you can tell *why* things are not going well. Is it a lack of clinical or procedural knowledge on your part? Are you struggling to make sense of what you are being told? Have you got all the information you need to assess the problem? Could it be that you haven't identified the 'right' problem, or, from the patient's point of view, are addressing the wrong one? Are you clear about which part of the consultation you are or should be in? Are you and the patient in the same part of the consultation; is the patient still trying to tell you their story while you have already moved on to management? Could you have made any wrong assumptions about the problem or committed the sin of premature medicalisation? Is there anything about your approach or your manner that might be upsetting the patient? Has your concentration lapsed because you have something else on your mind? If this is an SCA case, has the fact that your performance is going to be watched and assessed got you flustered?

Think aloud: In another of those two-part steers I'm so keen on, explain what the difficulty is and what would help. So you could say, 'I'm sorry, I've realised I don't know enough about this. I'd like to check something in a reference book.' Or, 'I don't think I've quite understood why this is such a worry for you. Tell me again what your main concern is.' Or, 'I'm afraid I've lost the thread of what I was going to say. Can you give me a moment to collect my thoughts?' As is usually the case when you think aloud, the patient's response will be to try and help, or at least will be sympathetic.[12]

'Take 2': Rewind and resume the consultation as near as possible from the last point, it was going well – this time, fingers crossed, more successfully.

Housekeeping: Lapses and dysfunctional moments like these are inevitably unsettling. Afterwards, do whatever is necessary to clear your

---

[12] In the SCA, even if it is imagining the examiner that has got you flustered, you should stay in role and still address your thinking aloud to the patient, e.g. 'Sorry, I've got myself in a muddle.' Don't try to explain to the examiner.

head and regain composure before seeing your next patient. Take comfort in knowing that the episode will have worried you much more that it will the patient. You might even see the funny side of it. Have a glass of water; take a short break; tell someone about it. Make a note of anything you need to look up to plug a knowledge gap.

If a 'wish-the-floor-would-open' moment happens during the SCA, do not despair. They tend to occur during the 'management' part of the consultation, either through clinical uncertainty or running short of time. If you don't know the right thing to do, do what you would do in real life – make a plan to find out. If your 12 minutes are about to run out before you have covered everything you intended to, quickly summarise what you would have done had there been more time. This way, it is still possible to score 1 or 2 of the 3 marks available and, if you have earned 5 or 6 already for data gathering and interpersonal skills, to gain a passing mark for the station.

Remote (telephone and video) consultations

Consultations by telephone are increasingly common in general practice; by 2019, they were accounting for about 25% of doctor–patient contacts in the United Kingdom. Consultation by video (computer, tablet or smartphone) has lagged some years behind, but remote consultations by phone and video both became far more widespread during the Coronavirus pandemic of 2020–2022, when face-to-face consulting carried a high risk. And of course, during the SCA, *all* your consultations will be either video or telephone ones. As I write, it is hard to predict where the balance between the various platforms will lie in post-pandemic general practice, but we can be confident of two things: (i) telephone and video will be more extensively used for triage and for low-risk or routine consultations, and (ii) patients will continue to present complex and sensitive problems where there is no substitute for the intimacy and thoroughness of a personal meeting with a doctor.

In essence, consultations by phone or video should follow the same structure as a face-to-face one, i.e. beginning with getting the patient's account of the problem as fully as possible, then obtaining all the information needed to assess it medically, and finally having the discussion from which an agreed plan of action can emerge. However, the limitations of phone and video as methods of communication mean that some compromises have to be made and some additional precautions taken. The obvious ones are that physical examination is impossible, and the exchange of visual information is non-existent by phone and significantly restricted even on video. These constraints increase the risk of misdiagnosis and of misinterpreting what the patient is trying to communicate.

Consulting by telephone

Telephone consultations tend to be more doctor-centred than usual; to focus more on the physical aspects of a problem than on its psychological, emotional and social components; and to risk underestimating the seriousness of a patient's symptoms. Why?

Firstly, GPs have become used to consulting by phone; to them, it is nothing special. But to many patients, anything other than seeing the doctor face to face is unfamiliar, leading them to adopt a more passive role in the consultation. Secondly, it's hard to show empathy over the phone. Many of the cues that help us recognise what another person is thinking and feeling – facial expression, body language, subtleties of language and tone of voice – are lost when the interaction takes place over a poor-quality audio channel. Finally, alert to the dangers of not being able to conduct a physical examination and rightly making patient safety their first priority, doctors have become very good at checking for red flag symptoms in the patient's narrative. But this can result in the phenomenon of 'cognitive bias,' where shortcuts in our thinking can lead to error. It is easy to assume that *If there are no red flags, the problem must be minor;* that *If I don't pick up any cues to emotional or psychological factors, there can't be any*; and that *Telephone consultations are meant for non-serious problems; this is a telephone consultation, so it can't be serious.*

Recognising the inherent shortcomings of telephone consultations goes a long way towards overcoming them. But there are some additional safeguards that can be grafted onto the usual consultation process.

- Familiarise yourself with the patient's records – past and recent history, medication, correspondence, path results, etc. – before making the phone call.

- Introduce yourself by name, and confirm the identity of the person you are speaking to. If it's not the patient, e.g. a parent, relative or carer, there may be issues of consent or confidentiality.

- Check where the patient is located. They may not be at their registered address, and this could be relevant if they need to be seen.

- If you have been given advance information about the reason for the call, e.g. by whoever triaged the original request, don't assume that what you have been told is the whole story. The next section explains more about this potential pitfall.

- Normally, during the Patient's part of a face-to-face consultation, we show we are listening and paying attention, and regulate the flow of conversation, by verbal and non-verbal signals called *pacing cues*. These include nodding, widening the eyes, noises like 'uh huh' and 'mmm,' and words like 'right' or 'OK.' On a phone line, the non-verbal cues are lost, and the 'uh-huh's and 'OK's can feel to the patient like inter-ruptions rather than encouragement. Try to reduce the number of ver-bal pacing cues, and make them more explicit when you do use them, so that they become more like proper receipts. So instead of murmur-ing 'Mmm … right,' say something like, 'I'm still listening, please go on,' or 'That's interesting, tell me more.'

- Be extra alert to possible indications of how the patient is feeling from the words they use and their tone of voice. If you think you hear evi-dence of some emotion, try a tentative receipt such as, 'It sounds like you're pretty worried,' or, 'I get the feeling you're a bit cross.'

- The inability to examine the patient cannot be overcome. Unless the patient has the necessary equipment, such as a sphygmomanometer or glucometer, asking the patient to self-examine and report the find-ings is hopelessly unreliable – even such apparently simple things as describing a rash or counting the pulse rate. Have a low threshold for arranging a face-to-face consultation. If you need to examine the patient, you need to examine the patient.

- Before finishing, summarise the consultation's main points, and ask the patient if they have any questions or if there is anything they would like you to explain again. Allow them time to think before they answer.

- Safety-netting is particularly important if you have not been able to examine the patient. Be explicit about what the patient is to expect, what to look out for that would suggest a need to consult again, and what they should do in that event.

- End with a friendly sign-off, such as, 'I've enjoyed talking to you. I hope that's been helpful.'

Don't rely on the triage information

Along with the rise in remote consulting as a result of the pandemic, there have been changes in the process whereby patients' requests for consulta-tions are triaged, to try to ensure that the patient speaks to or is seen by the health-care professional deemed most appropriate. This more comprehen-sive triage, although inevitable, carries some risks.

In the 'old' pre-COVID days, a patient wanting to see a doctor would negotiate an appointment with a receptionist, either by phone or in person. The receptionist would probably ask for enough information to determine the degree of urgency, but would not ask – nor would the patient think it appro-priate to *be* asked – for intimate personal details of the symptoms or problem.

However, even before the pandemic, some practices were adopting sys-tems of 'total triage,' a trend that accelerated once face–to–face consultations ceased to be the norm. Triaging patients' requests was no longer a simple matter of deciding 'which doctor and when'. At the patient's first point of contact with the Surgery, a decision had to be made as to which professional should deal with them — doctor, nurse, nurse practitioner, physician associate, community pharmacist … — and what was the appropriate format or location — a telephone call, a face-to-face appointment, the NHS 111 Helpline or direct referral to a hospital A&E department. All this complexity required the patient to disclose far more details of their problem than had hitherto been the case. And that disclosure might have to be made not just to a known receptionist but to an anonymous voice, or as a recorded message, or to an on-screen algorithm or chatbot, or on an email proforma.

Many patients were uneasy at the extent of self-revelation being required of them by a triage system whose security and confidentiality they had no way of judging. As a result, some were guarded, tending to downplay their symptoms or describe their problem only in vague terms. Others, determined to get past what they saw as an unwelcome obstacle, would exaggerate their problem in language that would fast-track them to the clinician of their choice. Thus a child's mild nausea might be reported as 'projectile vomiting', or muscular stiffness after gardening as 'chest pain on exercise'.

The message for a GP embarking on a series of telephone consultations and armed with a list giving the supposed reason for each call is: 'You cannot rely on the triage information.' It may or may not be accurate or complete; to assume that the problem as stated at triage is the *real* problem risks making wrong assumptions and closing one's mind to other possibilities.

For example, a woman with a vaginal discharge she thinks may be a sexually transmitted infection caught from her adulterous husband is highly unlikely to explain her worries at the triage stage. Instead, she will probably say she thinks she has a urine infection. Taken at face value, this information will probably result in her being given an inappropriate antibiotic prescription without being seen. If she does receive a telephone call from a doctor and the doctor begins by saying, 'I gather you have cystitis', the consultation is already off to a dysfunctional start and may end up addressing the wrong problem. It's better, I think, to start a telephone consultation just as you would a face-to-face one, with an open-ended 'How can I help?' If the patient, irritated, replies, 'I've already explained that; haven't you read the message?' I recommend a soothing 'Yes, but I'd really like you to tell me about it in your words, to make sure I understand properly.'

Consulting by video

Much of what I have said about telephone consultations also applies to video. Being able to see each other undoubtedly increases the amount of information exchanged between doctor and patient. But the more complex technology raises some additional issues.

Conversing by video is commonplace amongst the IT-literate popula-tion, but much less so for people who are poor, elderly or socially disad-vantaged. There is a danger that a greater prevalence of technologically sophisticated forms of consulting could further increase the United Kingdom's already regrettable health inequalities.

You will probably conduct your video consultations in a quiet, well-lit room, using a desktop or laptop computer. Your patient, however, may be using a hand-held tablet or smartphone in a noisy environment with uncertain privacy. With most video platforms, moreover, the bandwidth and stability of the internet connection limit the quality of the picture and can cause it to jerk or sometimes freeze. Or it may introduce a small time delay or cause picture and sound to be out of sync. These distractions all make it easier to miss significant information. So:

- If video consulting is to be a regular part of your practice, see if it is possible for patients new to the format to be given some prior informa-tion, perhaps by a receptionist, about how it works and what to expect.

- If you are video-consulting from home, choose a neutral setting and background, so that the patient is not distracted by glimpses of your domestic circumstances. Dress professionally. Make sure you will not be interrupted and that background sounds are not intrusive.

- Give some thought to how your image will look on the patient's screen. Landscape format feels more natural than portrait. Hand gestures are an important part of communication; adjust your distance from the camera so that the patient can see your hands as well as your face. Make sure your face is well lit, and avoid having a source of bright light behind you.

- At the start of the consultation, before you get on to the patient's prob-lem, ask for a phone number where you can call the patient if the video link proves unsustainable.

- Time lags between one of you speaking and the other hearing what has been said are more common over a video link. This means that pacing cues – the 'uh huh's and 'OK's – can be even more disruptive than they are over the phone. Convey your interest and attentiveness by eye contact and facial expression. (If you want to make eye contact with the patient, remember to look at the webcam, not the image of the patient's face on the screen.) If you need to interrupt the patient, try a visual signal, such as rais-ing your hand. Rapid gestures can be distracting; try to slow them down.

- Video-consulting, especially from home, can be lonely. Make sure you have the opportunity for a regular debrief with a colleague, where you can discuss clinical matters and also any feelings of stress or concern you may be experiencing.

E-consulting

Recent years have seen the development of an online consultation platform called eConsult, now increasingly available via the NHS app. eConsult allows patients to submit their symptoms or requests electronically to a practice, and, in return, receive some emailed information or advice, a prescription, a sick note, a phone call or face-to-face appointment – whatever the practice unilaterally decides is appropriate. While there are undoubted advantages to e-consulting on straightforward or administrative issues (if you have the necessary technology), the absence of real-time interaction between patient and doctor places the process outside consulting, as I understand it. In an e-consultation, data-gathering is structured by the algorithm and thus almost entirely doctor-led, with only a minimal Patient's part and absolutely no possibility of shared decision-making.

Luckily, the philosophy and politics of healthcare delivery are outside the scope of this book, or it would have been much longer.

Preparing for the SCA

EXAM POINT: Content of the SCA exam

Although specific case scenarios will be different for each session of the SCA, the college has indicated in webinars that the following clinical areas are likely to be covered each time:

- a patient less than 19 years old;
- gender, reproductive and sexual health, including women's, men's, LGBTQ, gynae and breast;
- long-term condition including cancer, multi-morbidity and disability;
- older adults, including frailty and people at the end of life;
- mental health, including addiction, alcohol and substance misuse;
- urgent and unscheduled care;
- health disadvantages and vulnerabilities, including veterans, mental capacity, safeguarding and communication difficulties;
- ethnicity, culture, diversity and inclusivity;
- new presentation of undifferentiated disease;
- prescribing;
- investigation / results;
- professional conversations and dilemmas.

In this section, I want to address two questions that worried SCA candidates frequently ask:

1   How can I cover everything in 12 minutes?
      and
2   What is the best way to prepare for the exam?

On both issues, it helps to be clear what the examiners are and are *not* looking for.

According to the RCGP, the purpose of the SCA is 'to assess the GP trainee's ability to integrate and apply clinical, professional and communication skills appropriate for general practice, whilst demonstrating and achieving the underlying principles of good medical practice in that:

- patients are kept safe;
- GPs can be adaptable in treating different types of patients and illnesses;
- GPs can manage risk, medical complexity and uncertainty; and
- GPs exhibit appropriate behaviours, attitudes and concerns for their patients.'

Translated out of committee-speak, this means, 'Show us that your clinical and communication skills are good enough for you to deliver safe, acceptably competent, personalised care as an independent GP in the NHS?'

In other words, the examiners want to see whether you can do what an ordinary British GP could reasonably be expected to do under everyday working conditions and without anybody holding your hand.

The examiners, who are all working GPs themselves, are *not* looking for:

- perfection or miracles;
- an encyclopaedic knowledge of 'small print' medicine;
- a checklist of things they want you to do or say;
- any particular model of the consultation;
- consultation jargon;
- a chance to trick you or trap you.

The RCGP's Latin motto is *Cum scientia caritas*, which means roughly *kindness with competence*. Demonstrate both in your consultations, and you will have no difficulty passing the SCA.

Running short of time

Every SCA case has been extensively piloted during its development, and it is perfectly possible to do enough to gain full marks in 12 minutes. Nonetheless, one of the main causes of losing marks in an SCA case is running out of time, especially time to complete the management – in the language of this book, the Shared – part of the consultation. Common reasons for this are:

- a haphazard or inefficient structure to the consultation;
- spending too long on data-gathering;
- having to go back to ask questions you should have asked earlier;
- remembering questions you *think* you should have asked earlier, which don't actually matter much, but going back and asking them anyway;
- looking for non-existent traps you suspect the examiners have set for you;
- trying to do too much in a single consultation, not prioritising;
- being nervous of taking control of timing and moving the consultation on;
- putting off doing the hard part of the consultation;
- not keeping an eye on the clock;
- not being used to doing 12-minute consultations.

Here are some tips for avoiding these pitfalls.

- Practise a structure for your consultations, such as the one described in this book, until it becomes second nature, your usual default way of consulting.
- Trust yourself to 'shut up and listen' at the beginning of the Patient's part.
- Most cues to relevant agenda will come during the first 2 or 3 minutes. Make sure you don't miss them.
- Don't be scared of time-managing the consultation. Patient-centredness includes getting the job done in the time available.
- Use receipts, two-part steers and thinking aloud to steer the consultation if necessary.
- Summarise early (but not *too* early), and be prepared to re-summarise.
- If you think you might be missing something important, ask, 'Is there anything else on your mind that you haven't yet told me about?' or 'Is there anything more you think I should know in order to help you?'
- Don't put off the difficult part of the consultation. It won't go away.

- Aim to move on to the Shared part by 7 or 8 minutes.
- Don't apply to do the exam until you are regularly doing 10-minute consultations in your training practice.
- In your usual consulting room in your practice, have a clock in a position where you can easily see it, e.g. on the wall behind the patient's shoulder. Try to develop an idea of what 'five minutes into the consultation' feels like, or 'only three minutes go if this was the SCA.'

EXAM POINT: Setting the SCA pass mark

All candidates sitting a particular session of the SCA will have the same 12 cases. But candidates sitting on another occasion will have a different 12 cases, which might be harder or easier. From the time of the CSA, the examiners have been at pains to ensure that the overall degree of difficulty of all 12 cases (the 'palette') is kept similar. For this reason, the pass mark for each sitting may vary slightly to reflect different degrees of challenge in individual cases. In semi-standardised assessments of this type, the internationally accepted way of setting the pass mark for the session is the borderline regression method.

In addition to marking a case with one of four grades (*Clear Pass, Pass, Fail* and *Clear Fail*) in each of the three marking domains, the examiner also records a global rating of the candidate's overall performance on the case. The borderline regression method takes all of every examiner's marks into account when determining the mark that is 'just good enough to deserve a pass' for each exam day.

Preparing for the exam

You can't bluff or play-act your way to success in the SCA (or indeed, to good practice in real life). It can't be said too often: the best way to prepare for the SCA is, in the weeks and months beforehand, to see lots of patients, get into good consulting habits such as those described in this book – and then, on the day, go into the exam and just do what you always do.

That said, there are some educational strategies that will help. The top two are:

1 Watch yourself on video
   and
2 No really, watch yourself on video.

I don't care if you hate it, or get embarrassed, or convince yourself that you consult much better when you're not being recorded. Get the camera out at least once a week and record a surgery. After one or two patients, you will lose your initial self-consciousness. You don't need to show the recording to anybody else or use any rating scales or evaluation checklists. Just watch yourself and your performance in private, as objectively as you can, and ask yourself questions like:

- What's it like to be a patient of this doctor?
- If I were in the patient's shoes, what would I be thinking and feeling?
- How would the patient describe the consultation afterwards?
- Do I seem to know what I'm doing?
- How much of the time am I talking? How much listening?
- Does the consultation seem to have a structure? And a sense of flow?
- At any given moment, is it clear what part of the consultation I'm in?
- Do I seem genuinely interested, or are some of my questions formulaic?
- Have I got any irritating mannerisms?
- What advice would I give this doctor (who happens to be me)?

Cultivating good attention

An effective way to develop the mindset of 'attentive curiosity' that gets the consultation off to a good start is as follows: Before you start a surgery, put a blank sheet of paper on the desk. After each consultation, as soon as the patient has left, write down what their first words were when they entered the room, 10 minutes or so earlier. You can only do this if you have remembered what they said, and you can only remember if you were paying attention at the time. So even only *having the intention* to write the words down later has the effect of heightening your attention.

Practising two-part steers

Write the words *Two-part steer* on a Post-it note or similar, and put it on your desk to remind you. Promise yourself that, at least once during every consultation, you will try to do a two-part steer – acknowledge something the patient has said with a receipt, and follow it by saying something that moves the consultation on: 'Thank you for telling me *that*; now let's talk about *this*.' You can't fail at this exercise; no one will know if you forget. But within a few days, you will have done it scores of times and will have become quite adept.

Developing confidence in thinking aloud

Do the same with thinking aloud. Put a reminder on your desk and see whether, once in each consultation, you can find an opportunity to tell your patient something of what you yourself are thinking or feeling that ordinarily you would have kept to yourself. This way, you can experiment with pushing the boundaries of your reticence and test the usefulness of 'calculated self-disclosure.'

Books and courses

Perhaps unsurprisingly with an expensive high-stakes assessment, there is an abundance of 'crammer' books and courses purporting to offer shortcuts to SCA success. Some were even being advertised before the exam's format was decided! In my opinion, you should beware of any that are not written or tutored by real examiners or others specifically sanctioned by the RCGP. Much of the material produced by outsiders gives a misleading idea of what is required to pass, e.g. unrealistically long lists of what 'the good candidate' will say or do, and inappropriate suggestions as to what jargon and clichéd phrases will impress the examiners. The RCGP website has a section of advice on *Preparing for the SCA*, and you can have confidence in any preparation courses organised by the College and its local Faculties.

Study groups

In many parts of the country, there are informal study groups where candidates can practise role-plays and provide mutual encouragement and support. Books of sample cases are useful sources of practice scenarios, but be wary of using them as the gold standard for model answers, for the reasons given above. Ideally, obtain the services of an experienced trainer or examiner as a moderator. Failing this, feedback from your colleagues, especially from the role-play patient, is particularly valuable.

How trainers can help

As the date of the SCA approaches (though not so far ahead that it dominates everything else), trainers can help by regularly offering exam-oriented feedback on some of their trainees' video-recorded consultations. It is important for trainers to be fully and correctly informed about the format and methodology of the SCA. They should therefore ensure that they are thoroughly familiar with all the information on the RCGP website, https://www.rcgp.org.uk/mrcgp-exams/simulated-consultation-assessment. When reviewing and discussing a trainee's consultation, the trainer should structure their comments around the SCA's three marking domains and the guidance (on the website) as to how marks are allotted within each domain.

The website includes a selection of video clips of sample cases, together with suggestions as to how these can be used in preparation (https://www.rcgp.org.uk/mrcgp-exams/simulated-consultation-assessment/case-content-sample). Watching these together could usefully form the basis for some planned tutorials. The College and some of its regional Faculties offer training seminars and webinars to help trainers get up to speed with the new assessment.

Trainers can also help by:

- ensuring trainees see a wide range of acute and chronic conditions and patient demographics;
- encouraging trainees to get used to video-recording their consultations;
- letting trainees sit in during some of their own consultations.

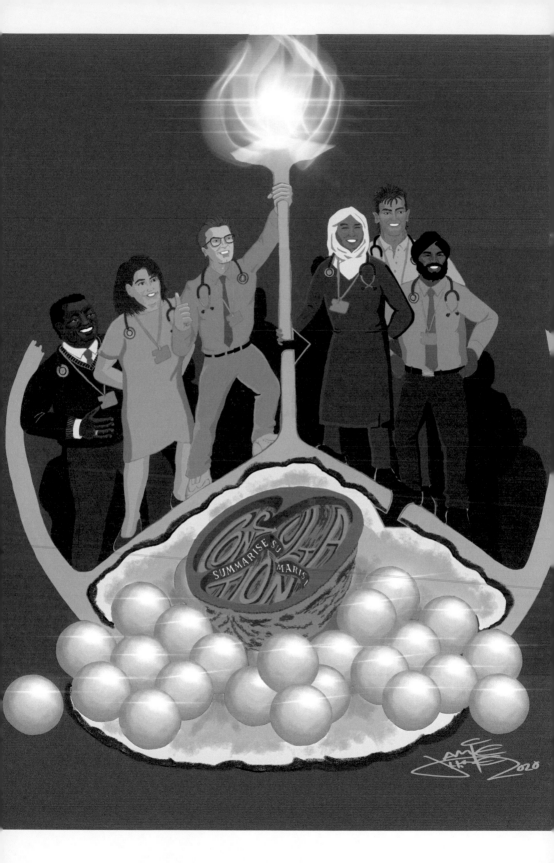

6

Before you go ...

... let me tell you the story of a young man who, as a boy, had a wonderful family doctor. Everyone agreed; they all said, 'She's a wonderful doctor.' You felt better just for seeing her, for knowing you were in her care.

In due course, the young man applied to medical school. He got all the right A-levels, played the clarinet and did the Duke of Edinburgh's Award, and told the selectors how he loved science but wanted to work with people. 'Just the sort of person we're looking for,' said the selectors. But really what drove him on was to be, in his turn, a wonderful doctor.

As the end of his medical studies approached, shortly before he was due to graduate, an admiring friend remarked on how much he must have learned in the last five years. 'That's true,' said the young man. 'I've been taught the causes and treatment of every condition. I've learned how to take a history and conduct an examination. I make sure I'm thorough, and logical, and up to date. And I've been taught how to communicate and encouraged to treat my patients as equal partners in their own health care.' But, he said, 'I keep thinking – when is someone going to teach me how to be wonderful?'

★ ★ ★ ★ ★

I won't claim that this or any other book can teach anybody to be a wonderful doctor. All I *will* claim for this book is that it sets out a simple structure as the basis for an effective and mutually satisfying problem-solving conversation between GP and patient. Yet not everyone will agree that even this is a good idea.

The danger of any simple account of a complex skill is that it can mislead beginners into thinking that mastery lies in following it slavishly, while more experienced practitioners wince at its very simplicity. Where is subtlety? they ask. Where is nuance? Individuality? Flair?

DOI: 10.1201/9781032619200-6

Fair points to all. So let me defend the importance of structure in competent consulting. Structure is not the enemy of flair, any more than grammar is the enemy of literature. Without a core of structure to give it shape and direction, a consultation is in danger of collapsing into gossip and guesswork. Without structure, flair is just flamboyance, and helpfulness just good intentions. For people early in their general practice careers, having an easy-to-grasp framework gives them courage, a first foothold on a difficult but rewarding climb. For those more worldly wise, structure is like the grain of sand in the oyster – the nugget of grit that, overlaid by layers of experience, grows to a pearl.

I hope this book, while explicitly addressed to specialist trainees in general practice with the SCA looming, will also be helpful to doctors both at the outset and in the heydays of their medical careers. We know that GPs' consultation styles evolve over time and that the consulting skills of new recruits to the profession are still work in progress. In most cases, they continue to mature, gaining in confidence, fluency and elegance. But a small minority of colleagues are like a pole vaulter having an off day; they clear the qualifying height but thereafter fall back, their consultations lapsing into something more doctor-centred, brusque and ultimately unsatisfying. The patients of such a doctor will seldom come to actual physical harm. But neither will they benefit from the myriad other ways in which more compassionate care could have helped them. Nor will those doctors come to appreciate the power and poignancy of the stories in which they themselves are characters.

All of which is my plea, at a time when general practice itself is rapidly evolving under the influence of technological advances and shifting social pressures, for us as professional generalists to continue to take pride in how we consult. In 2019, the *British Journal of General Practice* published an article of mine[1] urging us not to be seduced away from delivering the personalised care which is our best insurance against general practice becoming a footnote in the history of medicine. In it, I wrote:

> Consulting skills are not a set of circus tricks, like spinning plates or lion taming. They are the expression, in words and behaviour, of our professional values. The consultation is a shop window where we display what we think is important about doctoring. To the patient, it is the litmus test of whether or not we in fact care as much as we say we do.

I hope you agree. And I hope your time in general practice brings you as much delight as mine did to me. Thank you for allowing me into your thoughts.

---

[1] Neighbour R. (2019) Yesterday's man? BJGP, 69(686): 456–457.

Index

Note: Page numbers in *italics* indicate figures in text.